AF567126

TRAUMA AND PREGNANCY

Edited by

Christine E. Haycock

PSG PUBLISHING COMPANY, INC.
LITTLETON, MASSACHUSETTS

Library of Congress Cataloging in Publication Data

Main entry under title:

Trauma and pregnancy.

Includes bibliographies and index.
1. Pregnant women--Wounds and injuries. 2. Fetus--Wounds and injuries. 3. Surgical emergencies.
I. Haycock, Christine E. [DNLM: 1. Pregnancy Complications. 2. Wounds and Injuries--complications.
WO 700 T7745]
RG580.W68T73 1985 618.3 84-19070
ISBN 0-88416-467-5

Published by:
PSG PUBLISHING COMPANY, INC.
545 Great Road
Littleton, Massachusetts 01460

Printed in the United States of America

International Standard Book Number: 0-88416-467-5

Library of Congress Catalog Card Number: 84-19070

To the growing number of surgeons who have dedicated their skills to the salvage of the traumatized patient.

CONTRIBUTORS

MARLENE J. ADRIAN, PhD
Professor and
Director, Biomechanics Research Laboratory
University of Illinois at Urbana-Champaign
Urbana, Illinois

HABIB ANWAR, MD FACIP
Formerly Instructor of Surgery
UMDNJ-New Jersey Medical School
Presently
San Diego, California

MOLLY S. CHATTERJEE, MD FACOG
Assistant Professor
Department of Obstetrics and Gynecology
Assistant Director, Maternal Fetal Medicine
UMDNJ-New Jersey Medical School
Newark, New Jersey

NICOLE COHEN-ADDAD, MD
Assistant Professor, Pediatrics
UMDNJ-New Jersey Medical School
Newark, New Jersey

ROGER W. COUNTEE, MD
Department of Neurosurgery
Lahey Clinic Medical Center
Burlington, Massachusetts

GAIL ELIOT, MD
Associate Professor of Clinical Radiology
UMDNJ-New Jersey Medical School
Newark, New Jersey

MAKRAM ERIAN, MD
Assistant Professor of Anesthesiology
Director of Obstetrical Anesthesia
UMDNJ-New Jersey Medical School
Newark, New Jersey

MANUEL FERNANDES, MD
Associate Professor of Surgery/Urology
UMDNJ-New Jersey Medical School
Newark, New Jersey

CHRISTINE E. HAYCOCK, MD
Associate Professor of Surgery
UMDNJ-New Jersey Medical School
Newark, New Jersey

GEORGE W. MACHIEDO, MD
Associate Professor of Surgery
UMDNJ-New Jersey Medical School
Newark, New Jersey

WILLIAM E. NEVILLE, MD
Professor of Surgery
Director of Thoracic Surgery
UMDNJ-New Jersey Medical School
Newark, New Jersey

DANDAMUDI V. RAO, PhD
Associate Professor of Radiology
UMDNJ-New Jersey Medical School
Newark, New Jersey

JOYCE M. ROCKO, MD
Associate Professor of Surgery
UMDNJ-New Jersey Medical School
Director, Emergency/Trauma Services
University Hospital
Newark, New Jersey

JOSEPH SEEBODE, MD
Professor and Chief
Section of Urology
UMDNJ-New Jersey Medical School
Newark, New Jersey

BUEL A. STAGGERS, MD PhD
Clinical Assistant Professor
Section of Orthopaedic Surgery
UMDNJ-New Jersey Medical School
Chief of Staff, Orthopaedic Unit
United Hospitals Medical Center
Newark, New Jersey

IRVING D. STRAUCHLER, MD
Clinical Assistant Professor of Surgery
UMDNJ-New Jersey Medical School
Newark, New Jersey

KENNETH G. SWAN, MD FACS
Professor of Surgery
Director of Section of General Surgery
UMDNJ-New Jersey Medical School
Newark, New Jersey

JAMES P. THOMPSON, MD
Associate Professor of Obstetrics and Gynecology
UMDNJ-New Jersey Medical School
Chairman, Department of Obstetrics and Gynecology and Maternal-Fetal Medicine
St. Joseph's Hospital and Medical Center
Patterson, New Jersey

WEN-HSIEN WU, MD MS
Professor and Chairman
Department of Anesthesiology
UMDNJ–New Jersey Medical School
Newark, New Jersey

ALEXANDER F. ZOLLI, MD
Assistant Professor of Surgery
Section of Cardiothoracic Surgery
UMDNJ–New Jersey Medical School
Newark, New Jersey

CONTENTS

FOREWORD

Christine Haycock is an unusual physician, and she has drawn together in these pages a unique volume of information illuminating a special area in trauma which should be and now is quickly available to all of those professionals in emergency rooms throughout the country who inevitably will have to deal with the traumatized pregnant patient and solve her special problems.

University Hospital of the University of Medicine and Dentistry of New Jersey has one of the busiest emergency rooms in the country, with 80,000 to 100,000 visits annually. Dr. Haycock and her colleagues have been thoroughly exposed to this vast patient population. As a former director of the emergency room and in her present position as Director of Surgical Ambulatory Services, Dr. Haycock comes naturally to her expertise and interest in trauma.

Dr. Haycock's talents are multifaceted. After completing training as a nurse, she gained admission to the State University of New York Downstate Medical School at a time when women required extra special abilities to gain this recognition. She entered full-time academic surgery in 1968 after completing her surgical training and a period in private practice. She has risen to a senior position on the attending staff at University Hospital and on the tenured faculty of UMDNJ–New Jersey Medical School. During this period, she has written widely in her two areas of major interest, trauma surgery and sports medicine. In the meantime, she found time to serve as president of the American Medical Women's Association, rise to the rank of Colonel in the Army Reserve, now commanding the 348th General Hospital, and be designated the Outstanding Woman

Physician in New Jersey by the state chapter of the AWMA in 1976.

I congratulate Dr. Haycock and her colleagues in this important work and anticipate it will find its way into every well structured emergency room in the country and be mandatory reading for those with a serious interest in trauma.

Benjamin F. Rush, Jr, MD
Professor and Chairman
Department of Surgery
UMDNJ–New Jersey Medical School
Newark, New Jersey

PREFACE

This book is intended for the general surgeon, the emergency medical specialist, and for any specialist who must manage the care of the traumatized pregnant patient.

Its purpose is to place in one volume the data required to provide specific information to aid the specialist in dealing with the additional problems pregnancy may present to the trauma physician.

The chapters have all been written by qualified experts in each specific area who have carefully researched the literature to augment their own personal experience.

University Hospital of the New Jersey Medical School, University of Medicine and Dentistry of New Jersey, is the major trauma center for northern New Jersey. A trained team of trauma residents headed by an attending surgeon is on duty 24 hours a day, so the experience of the authors is extensive in the field.

The last chapter, by Marlene Adrian of the University of Illinois, was written at my request. Dr. Adrian and I have worked together in the past on sports medicine research, and she is particularly interested in the pregnant athlete. I felt that this would provide a unique chapter to the book not usually found in trauma texts.

Dr. Chatterjee of our Department of Obstetrics and Gynecology has provided in concise fashion the first chapters on the physiology and general medical problems that might be encountered in the pregnant patient.

Since one would normally expect the surgeon to be working with the obstetrician, detailed information in this regard was felt to be unnecessary.

With the numbers of pregnant women increasing now that the baby boom generation is reaching reproductive age and violence unfortunately increasing in our lives, it is our hope that this book will find a useful place on the surgeon's shelf.

ACKNOWLEDGMENTS

The editor gratefully acknowledges the help and contributions of the following persons:

Stephen K. Murata, Editor of *Consultant Magazine*, who encouraged me to write my initial article on trauma and pregnancy, to Willy Kratil, who aided me with preparing the photography work, and to Margaret Crane, Willa Jackson, and Anita Patrick, who provided secretarial and computer services without which I would have been stranded.

I also thank Mrs. Esther Meiboom, our Librarian, who aided me with obtaining reference material from the George C. Smith Library of the University of Medicine and Dentistry of New Jersey–New Jersey Medical School, and I thank my colleagues at the Medical School, who aided and encouraged me in the preparation of the book.

Finally, I must acknowledge the patience and understanding of my husband, Sam Moskowitz, himself an author and editor of many books and two magazines, who provided editorial advice when asked and encouragement when it was needed.

CHAPTER 1

PHYSIOLOGY OF PREGNANCY

MOLLY S. CHATTERJEE

When one considers the rising numbers of statistics related to trauma in the United States, it becomes very obvious that the busy trauma surgeon at some point in his career is going to have to deal with injured pregnant patients. To do so, it is necessary for him to understand the physiologic changes that occur at the various stages of pregnancy.

It is, therefore, important with a text of this type that the initial chapter deal with the physiology and anatomy of pregnancy. Throughout the book every effort will be made to correlate the physiologic changes occurring in the three trimesters of pregnancy with the injury, especially in those chapters relating to various types of injury where the location of the uterus, the changes in volume, etc, may have a direct effect or importance in the treatment of these injuries.

In the first trimester of pregnancy the uterus sits deep in the pelvic cavity within a protective wall formed by the bony pelvis. The uterus enlarges slowly so it is not until approximately the third month or the second trimester that it actually rises above the bony protection. It is after this third month that the upper portion of the uterus becomes vulnerable to injuries such as blunt trauma. Along with the increase in the size of the uterus there is an enlargement of the vessels supplying the uterus, and as these become proportionately larger they are more vulnerable to severe hemorrhage with injury.

In addition to the uterus itself, the developing placenta acts as a new endocrine organ with an outpouring of protein and steroid substances which bring about multiple physiologic changes during the pregnancy. The placenta also functions as an arteriovenous shunt to bring forth changes in the maternal cardiovascular system. The normal weight gain in most women during pregnancy varies from 24 to 27.5 lb (ca. 10.9 to 12.5 kg). Weight gain beyond these usual amounts often leads to complications and, in the case of trauma, may make any surgery that may become necessary on the pregnant patient that much more difficult, as is true of any obese patient. To facilitate this discussion, let us take a look at a system review of the changes that may occur.

GASTROINTESTINAL SYSTEM

The gastrointestinal tract motility gradually diminishes with the increasing size of the uterus, and this may result in reflux esophagitis along with reduced acid secretion. Should the patient have had a previous hiatal hernia, it may cause an exacerbation of this problem. Abdominal distension and constipation are an increasingly common complaint in the later stages of pregnancy. Constipation is aggravated by increased water reabsorption. Cholestasis in the liver, gall bladder, and biliary tract may result in increased risks in the development of cholelithiasis, especially in patients who have their first pregnancies in their late teenage years.

This decreased gastrointestinal motility may make it difficult in diagnosing blunt intraabdominal injury as it will mimic the development of diminished gastrointestinal sounds due to trauma, and it may also lead to the false assumption that the decreased intestinal sounds are due to injury. This must be kept in mind. The possibility of cholelithiasis may cause right upper quadrant pain that could mistakenly be thought to be due to injury to the hepatic systems, whereas it may be merely an exacerbation of this disease.

RESPIRATORY SYSTEM

In general, the vital capacity of the lungs remains unchanged throughout pregnancy. The expiratory reserve and the residual volume, however, are diminished. Increased oxygen consumption is necessary because of the increased needs of the growing fetus and placenta, and this can result in a dyspnea that is due to the pregnancy itself. Again, this dyspnea can be a confusing symptom in the diagnosis of blunt injury, particularly where there may be thoracic problems. The respiratory rate increases and the tidal volume increases in normal patients, particularly toward the final stage of the pregnancy.

Hyperventilation due to a direct effect of the placental progesterone on the medullary respiratory center may occur and cause mild respiratory alkalosis. The functional residual capacity, which is a combination of residual volume and expiratory reserve, is diminished due to elevation and relative immobility of the diaphragm. The respiratory motions therefore become mainly thoracic rather than abdominal during pregnancy. Small airway function is unaffected during pregnancy as is shown by measurement of the maximum expiratory flow volume and airway closing capacity.

CARDIOVASCULAR SYSTEM

In discussing cardiovascular changes here, I will not go into any abnormalities as these are discussed later in the chapter. In general there has been a good deal of controversy in the literature about the changes in the cardiac output in pregnancy. Cardiac output rises during the first 10 weeks of pregnancy and reaches a peak at 24 weeks, and the rise is then generally maintained until term. The heart rate rises by 15 to 20 beats per minute; there is a small rise in stroke volume, and at mid trimester there is a drop in the diastolic pressure, which is a well-known phenomenon and should be kept in mind for the diagnosis of preeclampsia and chronic hypertension as well as in dealing with a traumatized patient. Peripheral resistance is considerably decreased during pregnancy, but the peripheral blood flow is greatly increased. Vascular dilation in the nasal mucous membrane is a frequent cause of bleeding of the nose in pregnant patients, and a very slight blow to the nose can cause quite a profuse hemorrhage.

The changes in the heart itself are probably due to the elevation of the diaphragm by the enlarging uterus. The heart is pushed up and rotated forward. The electrical axis deviates to the left, causing occasional depression of ST segments, and a deep wave in lead 3 is a common EKG finding. Grade I or II systolic murmurs may be frequent over the base of the heart and should always be differentiated from organic heart disease in pregnancy.

The plasma volume starts to increase by 10 weeks of pregnancy, and a plateau is reached by 34 weeks. The total increase is usually about 50%. In preeclampsia there is a smaller rise in the plasma volume. The erythrocyte volume increases by 18% starting in the 10- to 20-week period of pregnancy. Due to the disproportionate increase in plasma and erythrocyte volume there is a state of so-called "hemodilution of pregnancy." Hemoglobin and hematocrit fall from the average nonpregnant value, and serum iron falls below the mean value mainly in the last trimester of pregnancy. Supplemental doses of iron are commonly recommended during pregnancy. This drop must be carefully kept in mind when dealing with the traumatized patient. Blood viscosity falls during pregnancy, and there is a marked leukocytosis, which again can be very confusing. Serum sodium, potassium, magnesium, calcium, and chloride fall during pregnancy. Bicarbonate falls early in the pregnancy along with a fall of the PCO_2 which is probably in line with the changes that occur in the respiratory volume.

The total serum proteins fall at the expense of the albumin fraction. The globulin fraction rises except for the gamma globulin. As a result, the albumin/globulin ratio changes. Alpha fetoprotein aglycoprotein is produced by the fetal liver and yolk sac and is noticed in increasing amounts in the maternal serum as pregnancy proceeds. Several protein substances are produced by the placenta, and these are gaining increased attention in the literature. These are commonly designated as pregnancy specific proteins.

Serum fibrinogen in pregnancy increases, resulting in an increased erythrocyte sedimentation rate. Serum copper and ceruloplasmin increases. The bleeding and clotting time remain unchanged; fibrinogen degradation products, however, tend to rise. The serum concentration of urea, uric acid, and creatinine fall. Serum folate and vitamin B_{12} are also at a lower level than in nonpregnant patients. Pregnant patients are more insensitive to angiotension than nonpregnant women. The status is changed, however, in preeclampsia.

URINARY TRACT

The renal plasma flow in the kidneys increases 45% by the ninth week of pregnancy. This change is brought about by increased cardiac output and low renal resistance. The glomerular filtration rate increases by 50% about two weeks after conception. The filtration fraction diminishes in early pregnancy, but increases by the last trimester. The renal collecting system dilates during pregnancy and persists up to 12 weeks of pregnancy. Glycosuria in pregnancy may be encountered due to increased glomerular filtration rate and a reduction in tubular maximum for glocuse.

Aminoaciduria is increased in pregnancy with simultaneous reduction of many amino acids in plasma. Further discussion on the changes in the urinary tract will be found in Chapter 14.

SKIN

Hyperpigmentation is a common phenomenon during pregnancy and is mainly noted around the nipple, areolar area, umbilicus, axilla, vulva, and perineal areas. The linea nigra is a common finding during pregnancy. Chloasma is noticed on the forehead, cheeks, temples, and upper lip. Striae gravidarum, or stretch marks, are mainly seen on the breast or lower abdomen. Palmar erythema or spider angioma may be noticed from the early months of gestation and may increase throughout pregnancy. The changes in the skin again may cause some difficulty in diagnosis and may be mistaken for bruise marks in the traumatized patient.

ENDOCRINE GLANDS

The anterior lobe of the pituitary gland hypertrophies. Gonadotrophin levels, follicle-stimulating hormone, and luteinizing hormone are low, and prolactin concentration is markedly elevated. Adrenocorticotropic hormone and thyroid-stimulating hormone are diminished. There is an increased thyroid stimulating hormone response to thyroitoxin releasing hormone which is noticed during the second half of pregnancy in some studies. The growth hormone response is reduced to both hypoglycemia and arginine during the third trimester of pregnancy. Oxytoxcin and vasopressin probably remain unchanged.

ADRENAL GLAND

The thickness of the zone fasciculata is increased. The plasma cortisol concentration rises progressively due to a rise in cortisol binding globulin. The half-life of plasma cortisol is prolonged in pregnancy, and free cortisol and aldosterone secretion is increased.

PARATHRYOID

The total serum calcium concentration falls in the serum progressively from 8 weeks of gestation, and the peak is reached between 28 to 32 weeks of gestation. Ionized calcium concentration remains unchanged during pregnancy. The parathyroid glands hypertrophy during pregnancy, resulting in increased parahormone levels. Calcitonin concentration probably also increases. The 1,2,5-dihydroxy vitamin D is elevated at term.

THYROID

Because of the increased estrogen production in pregnancy, thyroxine-binding globulin increases. The thyroid gland enlarges, and the basal metabolic rate rises. Radioactive iodine thyroid gland uptake also increases. Total thyroxine increases, and 3,5,3-triiodthyronine and resin uptake is diminished. The free thryoxine and 3,5,3-triiodythyronine remain unchanged.

PLACENTA

The placenta serves as an endocrine organ along with its other functions. Basically, it produces two kinds of hormones: the steroids and the polypeptides. The steroid hormones are progesterone, estradiol, estrone, and estriol. The main protein hormones of the placenta are human chorionic gonadotropin and human placental lactogen. The enzymes produced by the placenta are insulinase, oxytocinase, diamine-oxidase, and heat-stable alkaline phosphatase. The pregnancy associated plasma proteins like PAPP-A, PAPP-B, and PSBG have unknown biological functions and are being evaluated at many centers worldwide.

This has been a brief overview of the main physiologic changes in the normal pregnancy. Additional changes will be discussed in the specialized chapters.

SELECTED READINGS

1. Bruce NW: Gestational adaption: Major systems, in Iffy L, Kaminetzky H (eds): *Principles and Practice of Obstetrics and Perinatology*, vol 1. New York, John Wiley & Sons, 1981, pp 671–701.
2. Hytten FE, Lind T: *Diagnostic Indices in Pregnancy*, Ciba-Geigy, 1975.
3. Pritchard J, Macdonald P: Maternal adaption of pregnancy, in *William's Obstetrics*, 16th ed. New York, Appleton Century Crofts, 1980, pp 221–259.
4. Tulchinsky D, Ryan K: *Maternal Fetal Endocrinology*. Philadelphia, The WB Saunders Co, 1980.

CHAPTER 2

MEDICAL PROBLEMS OF THE PREGNANT PATIENT

MOLLY S. CHATTERJEE
CHRISTINE E. HAYCOCK

Since it is always possible that the injured pregnant patient may also be suffering a medical problem during her pregnancy, a brief review of the major problems that may be encountered follows.

TOXEMIA OF PREGNANCY

Toxemia is probably a misnomer, as no "toxin" has ever been isolated in this disorder of pregnancy. Hypertension, edema, proteinuria, and occasional convulsions are the manifestations of the disease. The American College of Obstetrics and Gynecology's classification of pregnancy induced hypertension is illustrated in Table 2-1.

Pathology of Toxemia

Initially, vascular resistance increases, leading to hypertension. The cardiac output may fall with the development of hypertension. The secretion of renin increases by the afferent arteriole of the glomerulus, and dilation of the renal vasculature is maintained by two locally synthesized prostaglandins—PGI_2 and PGE_2. Renin secretion is influenced by the delivery of sodium to the maculadensa and the sympathetic nervous system. Renin is responsible for the synthesis of the potent vasopressor agent, angiotensin II an octapeptide from angioten-

Table 2-1
American College of Obstetrics and Gynecology–1972 Classification of Pregnancy Induced Hypertension

Mild gestational disorders
Gestational or transient hypertension
Gestational edema
Gestational proteinuria
Acute toxemia: preeclampsia and eclampsia
Chronic hypertensive disease of whatever cause
Chronic hypertension with superimposed preclampsia or eclampsia
Hypertensive disease with insufficient information to allow classification

sinogen and angiotensin I. Aldosterone secretion is stimulated by angiotensin II which, in turn, expands extracellular volume.[1]

Uterine blood flow is reduced in toxemia of pregnancy. As mentioned in Chapter 1, the angiotensin sensitivity increases in preeclampsia long before the clinical signs and symptoms appear. This is the basis of the positive "roll-over" test reported by Gant et al.[2] Edema may be present in 75% of normotensive women. But the presence of edema with hypertension is pathological and indicates sodium retention and subsequent increase in extracellular volume. In preeclampsia the glomerular filtration rate is diminished, causing sodium retention. The plasma volume is also diminished by 9%.

Fibrinogen, factors VII, VIII, X, and XIII increase in normal pregnancy with diminution of fibrinolytic activity. In preeclampsia, increased platelet aggregation has been noticed with the possibility of hypercoagulopathy. This phenomenon may be linked to PGI_2 synthesis.

Clinical Picture

The incidence of toxemia in pregnancy is about 7%. This is a disease most prevalent in young primigravida and older multiparous patients. A rise in systolic blood pressure by 30 mm Hg, or the diastolic by 15 mm Hg, the mean arterial pressure (diastolic + 1/3 pulse pressure) of 90 mm Hg, or an absolute figure of 140/90 mm of Hg is considered as evidence of toxemia along with edema, proteinuria (more than 300 mg in 24 hours), and excessive gain in weight (more than 2 lb [ca. 907 g] per week). Underlying essential hypertension or renal disease increases the incidence of toxemia. Examination of the fundus oculi may show arteriolar narrowing.[3]

Management of Toxemia

Although preeclampsia is not preventable, eclampsia is. Early diagnosis and bed rest with sedation (phenobarbital, 60 mg) is recommended for mild preeclampsia. The baseline hemoglobin, hematocrit, blood urea nitrogen, creatinine, and uric acid are determined, and a 24-hour urine protein and creatinine clearance is obtained. A daily weight check and frequent blood pressure and urine protein testing are carried out. If the patient is at term, prompt delivery is the treatment of choice.

In severe preeclampsia, parenteral magnesium sulfate is started to achieve a therapeutic level of 3 to 6 mg/L, and delivery is considered. Diuretics are condemned in preeclampsia. If the diastolic blood pressure is more than 110 mm Hg, hydralazine or methyldopa is the drug of choice. If eclampsia develops, $MgSO_4$ is the drug of choice, but diazepam (Valium) or sodium phenobarbital can be used judiciously.

Long-Term Effect of Toxemia

There is recurrence of toxemia in 50% of multiparous women and in 25% of primiparous patients. There is controversy in the data available as to what percentage of women suffer from hypertension or renal disease in later life as a result of this entity.

DIABETES IN PREGNANCY

Due to the physiologic changes, pregnancy is known to be diabetogenic. This is reportedly due to the alterations in carbohydrate metabolism. The fasting blood glucose level is lowered during pregnancy; there is controversy about data regarding insulin levels during pregnancy. High levels of free fatty acids, ketones, triglycerides, human placental lactogen, and cortisol are common during pregnancy and may be antagonistic to insulin action. This may also explain the so-called "insensitivity" to insulin characteristic of pregnancy. As mentioned in Chapter 1, glycosuria is common during pregnancy.

Glucose utilization is increased in pregnancy as a consequence of its uptake by the fetus. Alanine availability for maternal gluconeogenesis is also reduced due to its active transport to the fetus.

The modified White's classification is probably more useful for follow-up of pregnant diabetics (Table 2-2). Identification of class A or gestational diabetics is based on an abnormal three-hour, 100-g oral glucose tolerance test. The screening procedures for diabetes in pregnancy have changed in recent years. Blood

Table 2-2
Classification of Diabetes Mellitus in Pregnancy*

A	Chemical diabetes
B	Maturity onset (age over 20 years), duration under 10 years, no vascular lesions
C_1	Age 10 to 19 years at onset
C_2	10 to 19 years duration
D_1	Under age 10 years at onset
D_2	Over 20 years at onset
D_3	Benign retinopathy
D_4	Calcified vessels of legs
D_5	Hypertension
E	No longer sought
F	Nephropathy
G	Many failures
H	Cardiopathy
R	Proliferating retinopathy
T	Renal transplant

*Modified from White P: Pregnancy and diabetes, in Marbel A, White P, Bradley RF, et al (eds): *Joslin's Diabetes Mellitus*, ed 11. Philadelphia, Lea & Febiger, 1971.

sugar is measured one hour after the administration of 50 g of glucose. If the blood sugar value is more than 135 mg/100 mL of plasma, a three-hour glucose tolerance test is warranted. The diagnosis and management of pregnant diabetics should never be based on the results of urine testing only. Patients with a family history are usually screened during pregnancy for diabetes. The routine screening of all pregnant women is carried out at some centers.[4]

Effects of Pregnancy on Diabetes

In the early months, hypoglycemia may be noticed. A decreased response of the maternal tissues to insulin causes an increase in insulin requirements in pregnant diabetics starting from about the fifth month of the pregnancy. After delivery, insulin requirements are rapidly reduced to prepregnancy needs or below.

Effects of Diabetes on Pregnancy

With the advent of insulin and a team approach to the management of pregnant diabetics, the spontaneous abortion and infertility rate in the diabetic is the same as in the general population. However, development of hydramnios, hypertensive disorders of pregnancy-pyelonephritis indicate poor prognosis.

Fetal and Neonatal Complications

The incidence of intrauterine fetal death is still higher in diabetic gravidas. Congenital malformations involving the heart, and the nervous and skeletal systems are the major cause of perinatal mortality. Elevated hemoglobin A_1C in the first trimester has been found to correlate with increased incidence of congenital malformations. The importance of periconceptual metabolic control of pregnant diabetics is thus being realized. The infant of a diabetic mother may manifest neonatal morbidity as respiratory distress syndrome, macrosomia, hypoglycemia, hyperbilirubinemia or hypocalcemia.

Management

Diet and insulin are the two mainstays of treatment of diabetes in pregnancy. The diet should contain 30 to 35 kcal/kg of actual body weight; 30% to 40% or 150 g is provided by carbohydrate. The protein content is generally 125 g per day, and the remainder of the calories are provided by 60 to 80 g of fat. The total calories are divided as follows: 24% at breakfast, 30% at lunch, 33% at dinner, and 13% in snacks.

Blood glucose control may require hospitalization. The patient will require daily blood sugar samples obtained at 7:00 AM, 11:00 AM, 4:00 PM, 9:00 PM, and 2:00 AM, along with urine sugar and acetone testing. With the advent of the glucose reflectance colorimeter and better patient education, blood sugars may be monitored at home four times daily (fasting and 2 hours after each meal). In motivated patients, insulin pumps are being considered. The plasma glucose should be maintained at less than 100 mg/100 mL for fasting and 120 mg/100 mL for postprandial measurements as recommended by Coustan.[5]

Oral hypoglycemics are not recommended in pregnancy as they cross the placenta and worsen the status of already existing fetal hyperinsulinemia. Insulin is the drug of choice for pregnant diabetics. Regular and long-acting insulins are administered according to the daily blood sugar levels.

Timing and Management of Delivery

Baseline electrocardiogram, fundoscopy, and renal function studies are done at or after the first prenatal visit. Rigid blood sugar controls are achieved throughout pregnancy. Fetal growth and well being studies (serial nonstress test-oxytocin challenge test, serum estriols, and ultrasound scans) are done. Signs and symptoms of complications are watched for. At about 38 weeks of gestation, amniocentesis is done to establish fetal lung maturity as evidenced by presence of phosphatidylglycerol.

If the cervix is favorable, labor is induced by oxytocin stimulation and artificial rupture of the membranes. If the cervix is not ripe, prolonged induction is always avoided, and caesarean section is done. During the course of induction, the patients are kept fasting, and subcutaneous insulin is withheld. An intravenous solution is started with 1000 mL of 5% dextrose in water with 0.5 N saline and 10 units of regular insulin. A fasting blood glucose is drawn before starting the intravenous line, and the urine is checked for sugar and acetone. Two hourly blood and urine samples are drawn, and 100 to 125 mL of intravenous fluid is infused per hour. The maternal glucose level is kept at 60–100 mg/100 mL and the insulin dose is increased or decreased according to the blood sugar level. Follow-up is mandatory for such patients, as about 60% of class A diabetics become overt diabetics in 16 years.[6]

HYPERTENSION IN PREGNANCY

It is often impossible to differentiate between preeclampsia and essential hypertension unless it is known that the patient was hypertensive before pregnancy.

The use of antihypertensive agents during pregnancy in the chronic disease has been controversial, yet the patient needs to have her disease controlled, and superimposed preeclampsia must be prevented or ameliorated. Should such a patient now add trauma to her problems she will present her physician with a real dilemma requiring careful cooperation between the surgeon and internist.

The effect of antihypertensive drugs on the uteroplacental circulation must be carefully considered as to whether the blood pressure of a gravid patient should be reduced.

The traumatized pregnant patient whose blood pressure was high due to chronic disease may be mistakenly thought to be normotensive on initial examination if this possibility is not kept in mind and the patient's medical history is not obtained quickly.

The treatment of essential hypertension in pregnancy is as mentioned under toxemia primarily with methyldopa and hydralazine, although it should be kept in mind that the latter may cause tachycardia. Mild hypertension is best controlled by diet and other general measures. Should the traumatized patient require diuretics, these can be given, but careful electrolyte monitoring is required.[7]

RHEUMATIC HEART DISEASE

Although the incidence of rheumatic heart disease has declined over the past two decades, it is still possible to encounter the pregnant patient with a significant cardiac complication such as mitral stenosis.[8] It is also possible that patients with such complications may require surgery, including valve replacement, before or during pregnancy.[9] While the likelihood of encountering such a patient in a trauma situation is undoubtedly low, it should be mentioned.

Since pregnancy still poses a high risk to rheumatic heart disease, patients with mitral disease and especially with artificial valves, therapeutic abortion will require serious consideration when trauma is superimposed on the situation.[8]

CONGENITAL CARDIOVASCULAR DISEASE

The number of surviving patients who now reach childbearing age is steadily increasing. If the lesion has been completely repaired, this patient requires no special attention when trauma occurs, but if the lesion has been partially corrected, trauma would prove a very serious additional load in the already stressed heart. Again, abortion or caesarean section may need to be considered early.[9]

Patients with lesions such as coarctation of the aorta and a bicuspid aortic valve have dangerous hemodynamic changes in any event. The addition of a traumatic episode could well be fatal.[10,11]

In general then, traumatized pregnant patients with any history of cardiovascular disorders require very close and careful assessment of cardiovascular function and constant monitoring.

REFERENCES

1. Ferris FT: Toxemia and hypertension, in *Medical Complications During Pregnancy*. Philadelphia, The WB Saunders Co, 1982, Chapter 1.
2. Gant NF, Chand S, Worley RJ, et al: A clinical test used for predicting the development of acute hypertension in pregnancy. *Am J Obstet Gynecol* 1974; 120:1.
3. Chesley LC: Hypertension in pregnancy definitions, familial factors and remote prognosis. *Kidney Int* 1980;18:234.
4. Felig P, Coustan D: Diabetes mellitus, in *Medical Complications During Pregnancy*. Philadelphia, The WB Saunders Co, 1982, Chapter 2.
5. Coustan DR: Recent advances in the management of diabetic pregnant women. *Clin Perinatol* 1980;7:299.
6. Gabbe SG, et al: Management and outcome of pregnancy in diabetes mellitus, classes B to R. *Am J Obstet Gynecol* 1977; 129:723.
7. Davidson JM, Lindheimer MD: Hypertension in pregnancy, in Sciarra J (ed): *Gynecology and Obstetrics*. Philadelphia, Harper and Row, 1983.
8. Ueland K: Dangerous cardiovascular lesions in pregnancy, in Sciarra J (ed): *Gynecology and Obstetrics*, vol 3, Philadelphia, Harper and Row, 1983.
9. Becher RM: Intracardiac surgery in pregnancy. *Infect Surg* 1983;2(8): 593–595.
10. Deal K, Wooley CS: Coartation of the aorta and pregnancy. *Ann Intern Med* 1973;78:706.
11. Goodwin JF: Pregnancy and coarctation of the aorta. *Clin Obstet Gynecol* 1961;4:465.

CHAPTER 3

PREOPERATIVE MANAGEMENT OF SHOCK IN THE PREGNANT PATIENT

JOYCE M. ROCKO
KENNETH G. SWAN

Trauma continues to be a major cause of death in the United States today. The most current data indicate that it ranks as the third most common cause of death among all age groups and both sexes.[1] Among those under the age of 40 years it is the most common cause of death.[2] The motor vehicle remains the most frequent cause of death by trauma; the figure, about 55,000 deaths per year,[3] is relatively constant despite attempts to improve safety within the vehicle and upon the highway, measures to enforce the nationwide 55 mph speed limit, and an overall reduction in miles driven per motor vehicle operator. Paralleling these alarming statistics is that related to gunshot wounds. Approximately 30,000 people succumb to gunshot wounds each year in the United States,[4] and it is apparent that the figure is on the increase. All of these data bode poorly for the pregnant individual.

Pregnancy is relatively uncommon after the age of 40 years. Thus, the segment of the patient population most vulnerable to death by trauma includes the most commonly cited reproductive years for the Western woman, namely, 15 through 40. Not surprising, then, is the fact that injury and death by trauma is on the increase in the pregnant population, and that gunshot wounds as etiologic agents are closing the gap between that source of trauma and injury secondary to motor vehicular accidents.

This chapter deals with the critical period between the traumatic event and the operative solution of the cause of shock which resulted. This time period is hopefully minimized, depending upon the severity of shock and its preoperative management, to only minutes to a few hours.

Shock is defined in many ways, but a few commonly accepted criteria include the following: 1) an abnormally low systemic arterial pressure, as registered by the sphygmomanometer; 2) tachycardia; 3) tachypnea; 4) diaphoresis; 5) agitation and mental confusion (manifestations of hypoxia); 6) abnormal organ function, such as a low urinary output (less than 25 mL per hour). Shock remains, however, inadequate tissue perfusion.

The ABCs of trauma care apply to the pregnant victim of trauma much as they do to any other victim of injury. They identify the following as major initial areas of concern: 1) airway; 2) breathing; and 3) circulation. Thus such patients must have a secure airway whether it be by spontaneous respiration or through the spectrum of airway access to include cricothyroidotomy if necessary. The establishment of a patent airway allows for assessment of breathing, which again ranges from spontaneous to assisted, and its adequacy is reflected in the appearance of the patient's color, including skin and mucous membranes, as well as reflected by analysis of arterial blood gases. The adequacy of circulation is determined by a number of criteria. These include restoration to near normal, hopefully to normal, of systemic arterial pressure, pulse, respiratory rate, mentation, and urinary output.

External bleeding such as that resulting from an open fracture or traumatic amputation of an extremity must be addressed immediately and presumably has been addressed "in the field." Internal bleeding as a source for or cause of shock is best addressed in the treating facility.

Thoracic trauma, whether penetrating or blunt in nature, requires rapid assessment of the nature of the injury and its sequelae. Ausculation of the chest may reveal decreased breath sounds on one side. This finding implies pneumothorax, hemothorax, or hemopneumothorax. Regardless of which of the three conditions exists, tube thoracostomy is indicated on the involved side. Because of its size the lung is the organ most commonly injured in chest trauma, regardless of whether the source is penetrating or blunt. Axiomatic is the fact that the injured and collapsed lung continues to bleed from its point of injury in most (85%) cases. The blood that drains out of the tube thoracostomy is ideally suited for autotransfusion. This has special application to the pregnant patient, for whom careless administration of whole blood without consideration of the potential threat to the fetus as well as mother has serious concern.

Since maternal shock has such a deleterious effect upon the fetus,[5,6] regardless of the duration of the pregnancy, immediate steps to erase the cause of this result of trauma must be instituted.

The condition must be reversed. Two lives depend upon the promptness of resuscitation. In most cases shock will be from hypovolemia when trauma is the inciting event. Thus, the establishment of an adequate airway, arrest of hemorrhage, and maintenance of cardiac function must be accompanied by replenishment to near normal of the circulating blood volume. Intravenous access must be instituted immediately, and several routes to include both upper and lower extremities are essential. The rationale behind access via an upper and a lower extremity relates to the fact that traumatic internal hemorrhage may prevent an infusion from reaching the heart and thereby render it ineffective. For example, if the traumatic event damages the subclavian vein, infusion into an upper extremity vein on the ipsilateral side may result in the resuscitation fluid draining into the pleural cavity on that side. The resultant hydrothorax or hemothorax has obvious consequences, unfortunately, often recognized only retrospectively. These include 1) failure to replenish lost circulating blood volume; 2) compromise of respiratory function; and 3) failure to recognize the cause of the ineffective resuscitative efforts. For similar reasons an intravenous access route in the lower extremity in the presence of injury to pelvic veins or the inferior vena cava will have comparable complications.

The choice of intravenous fluid for resuscitation of a pregnant victim of trauma who is in shock is controversial. Uncontested however is the fact that shock threatens the fetus more than the mother.[7] Fetal hypoxia resulting from shock is the number one cause of death in trauma with respect to the fetus whose mother sustains injury. Most traumatologists favor initial resuscitation with lactated Ringer's solution and in a ratio (3:1) that well exceeds the estimated whole blood loss. Alternatives include saline and dextrose in water among many options in the crystalloid category. Ringer's lactate is preferred because it is "more physiologic." By that is meant the composition of electrolytes within the solution. Dextrose–water is free of essential electrolytes such as sodium, potassium chloride, etc., and thus is the least desirable of those solutions mentioned. So-called physiologic saline (0.9%) is in fact not physiologic since it contains 154 mEq of chloride per liter, which places it well above normal serum isoosmolar levels in man (chloride 100 mEq/L). Should relatively large volumes of saline be administered to the pregnant patient, she and her fetus, like any victim of trauma, may sustain the complications of hyperchloremic acidosis.

Should colloid be the treatment of hypovolemic shock in the pregnant patient? This question is controversial, and perhaps the best solution to the controversy is a compromise. Without indulging in the pros and cons to an unproductive end, we would favor initial resuscitation with crystalloid, consisting of Ringer's lactate solution, and where blood loss to a significant degree (more than 1000 mL in a patient less than 50 kg) is defined, administration of whole blood or its components.

The use of type-specific whole blood has won favor in most trauma circles when whole blood is required by a trauma victim. The time necessary for blood typing and replacement should be 5 minutes or less. In the Vietnam conflict the elapsed time was 22 seconds![4] In the pregnant patient the Rh antigen is a serious consideration, every effort should be expended to determine her positivity or negativity before blood infusion.[8] This consideration relates to implications of not only the current pregnancy but also possible future pregnancies. It is for this reason that blood type O with negative Rh antigen is probably the treatment of choice when time precludes the more optimal use of type-specific and cross-matched blood in obstetrical trauma care. Regardless of the theoretical approach to the obstetrical patient in shock, the shock must be corrected by whatever means at hand to anticipate fetal and maternal recovery after trauma.

Additional measures in resuscitation of the obstetrical patient of trauma include a thorough history and physical examination and intubation of both the stomach and the urinary bladder. The latter require nasogastric intubation and transurethral (Foley) catheterization. These tubes are both diagnostic and therapeutic in nature. There are obvious contraindications to their use, but in general, they are routine in the management of any victim of trauma, obstetrical or otherwise.

The history must include an obstetrical record, including previous pregnancies and their outcome, the date of the last menstrual period, dystocias, previous trauma, previous surgical procedures, hospitalizations, systemic illnesses, allergies, immunizations, current medications, and not to be minimized, any evidence of drug abuse or psychiatric disturbance. Detailed, if possible, information regarding these considerations is essential for the welfare of both mother and fetus when trauma is an in citing event leading to hospitalization. This information may be obtained from the patient or her relatives, even bystanders. Bystanders may be able to identify such essentials as the nature of the accident, its circumstances, and its outcome. If it was a motor vehicle accident, what was the speed, what were the impact point and site, were others injured, were seat belts worn, and were the chest and abdomen supported? Was fire a result of the accident? Remember, hypoxia is a significant threat to the mother and even more to her fetus. The treatment of both is oxygen, by whatever airway is instituted, and in high concentrations.

Carbon monoxide poisoning is a consequence of excessive thermal exposure, such as occurs during a fire. The metabolic half-life of carboxyhemoglobin, assuming respiration with sea level air, is about 2.5 hours, whereas with assisted ventilation and 100% oxygen, the time falls to about 30 minutes. These principles are crucial to salvage of both mother and fetus. Thus, while the history is being obtained, therapy must be instituted.

Physical examination will show the source and site of injury in most cases. The physician must examine for the source of shock, which in most cases may be external blood loss. The techniques of controlling hemorrhage include 1) direct digital pressure, 2) direct compression, 3) tourniquet, and 4) occlusion with vascular clamps of major vessels. Obviously, these techniques apply only to those sources of external hemorrhage which attend injuries to extremities, the head, and the neck. When shock is a result of internal hemorrhage, whether by blunt or penetrating trauma, the treatment is more problematic. If the injury is thoracic, then the principles of management of thoracic trauma apply. There are well-defined indications for tube thoracostomy and thoracotomy in the management of trauma victims, particularly those in shock and who will probably require operative intervention. For the obstetrical victim of trauma several considerations are pertinent to her management and that of her conceptus. If chest trauma is the source of shock then clinical observation is the important determining factor. Auscultation of the chest may reveal decreased breath sounds and by itself indicates tube thoracostomy on the involved side. Should doubt exist as to the clinical findings in support of pneumothorax, hemothorax, or hemopneumothorax, tube thoracostomy is still indicated. There should be negligible morbidity and mortality associated with tube thoracostomy in the hands of experienced traumatologists. Diagnostic thoracentesis is to be condemned. The indication of thoracentesis is the indication for tube thoracostomy. Even bilateral tube thoracostomy can be performed when doubt exists as to the degree of trauma to the chest.

Should the tube thoracostomy drain sufficient quantities of blood, the blood is ideally suited for autotransfusion. This blood is usually anticoagulated, is obviously typed and cross matched and, more importantly, is rapidly available for infusion. It is not likely to be contaminated by bacteria and can be easily administered with a hand pump and via a micropore filter to eliminate any debris that may accompany the drainage and infusion process. Rapid tube thoracostomy will save lives, and the pregnant patient is no exception, especially when one considers that two, not one, lives are at stake. Shock caused by hemothorax is usually due to pulmonary parenchymal injury when trauma is the insult. This relates to the fact that the lung is the largest target in the chest. Injury to the lung causes it to collapse. The collapsed lung continues to bleed; with mediastinal shift, a pleural cavity can accommodate up to 3 L of blood loss. Without replenishment, this loss is obviously poorly tolerated by even the most healthy adult. The rapid reexpansion of the lung on the injured side is essential for the successful resuscitation of all trauma victims, especially pregnant ones. There are numerous other indications for tube thoracostomy in the management of the trauma victim which are discussed in a subsequent chapter.

Should open thoracotomy be carried out when a pregnant patient arrives at the emergency room with a history of trauma and sudden, in transit, or observed death? The answer is yes. The pregnant patient who is subject to trauma does not differ from any other trauma victim. She deserves even more consideration since she includes an additional victim, the fetus she bears. Additionally, she is statistically relatively young and very resuscitatable. Thus, open thoracotomy is indicated even in the emergency room to address and control presumed injuries to the heart or great vessels. Radiography may assist in the diagnosis, but is often not available for logistic reasons. For the same reasons, radiographic identification of the nature of the trauma may be unsound clinically, since time is a factor, and time may be lost by undue radiographic investigation. The latter should not be a prerequisite for the definitive care of the trauma victim. Thus, open thoracotomy, whether through a left lateral or a median sternal approach, is always indicated when imminent demise is diagnosed. Injuries to the thoracic contents can be addressed appropriately. Space does not permit a detailed discussion of techniques. However, should a hole in the respiratory diaphragm be identified during thoracotomy, exploratory laparotomy is indicated. Intraabdominal injury is implied.

Since automobile accidents account for such a high percentage of obstetrical trauma,[9,10] the physician should be alerted to the possibility of myocardial contusion and rupture of the thoracic aorta as a cause of shock. The electrocardiogram will be of assistance as well as the chest roentgenogram in these determinations. Where doubt exists, angiography to include aortic arch studies is indicated. Recall that the well being of the fetus is dependent upon maternal welfare, and thus the threat of radiational hazard to the fetus must take secondary consideration to the diagnosis and therapy of the mother's injury.

Hemopericardium and pericardial tamponade may attend any victim of trauma and must be diagnosed as rapidly as possible. Beck's triad of 1) distal heart sounds on auscultation of the pericardium; 2) systemic venous hypertension and 3) systemic arterial hypotension are clues to pericardial tamponade. The latter is an ominous and near-fatal recognition. In any event the suspicion of pericardial tamponade is an indication for thoracotomy in the emergency room. The patient is suffering from shock and requires immediate evacuation of the pericardial contents. Often as little as 30 mL of blood will restore the patient's vital signs to near normal. The latter procedure can be accomplished, if necessary, enroute to the operating room, where the definitive control of a myocardial injury can be better addressed.

More commonly, the pregnant victim of trauma has sustained abdominal trauma whether by blunt or penetrating source. Regardless of the cause of the trauma, the approach should be the same. History has been discussed. Physical examination is also important, especially with regard to the abdomen. The hallmark of abdominal trauma is pain and tenderness. These two findings imply peritonitis. The latter can occur as a result of blood alone in the peritoneal cavity. The exact mechanism whereby blood induces peritoneal irritation is an enigma. Nonetheless, the findings of an "acute abdomen" coupled with a history of trauma should alert the physician to the need for exploratory laparotomy. The pregnant patient is no exception to this rule. Her survival and that of her fetus is dependent upon prompt identification of the source of bleeding within the peritoneal cavity and its resolution. Regardless of the length of gestation, the treatment is the same, and its purpose is to control hemorrhage that will culminate in shock.

Most surgeons would agree that evidence of peritoneal penetration by whatever traumatic event is an indication for exploratory laparotomy. The definition of implied peritoneal penetration can be based upon history (eg, a gunshot wound), physical findings (an acute abdomen), laboratory determinations such as a positive peritoneal lavage (greater than 100,000 erythrocytes per mm^3 or more than 500 leukocytes per mm^3 of lavage return), or radiographic observations such as gas under the respiratory diaphragm, intravenous pyelographic evidence of injury to a kidney or its ureter, or cysto-urethrographic evidence of injury to the bladder or urethra. All of these findings suggest the need for abdominal exploration. But when doubt exists as to the possible injury to intraabdominal viscera there should be no hesitation on the part of the surgeon to examine operatively the intraabdominal contents. The gravid patient is no exception to this axiom. Length of gestation is a consideration, but never a contraindication to exploratory laparotomy.

A review of the above observations is germane to the decision to operate to interdict life-threatening hemorrhage and shock. The very high incidence of surgically significant intraabdominal injury associated with gunshot wounds to the abdomen[11] makes that observation alone an indication for exploratory laparotomy regardless of the duration of gestation. Injury to the abdomen by pointed instrument carries a lesser incidence of surgically significant intraabdominal pathology.[5] Thus, additional assessment is appropriate. Statistically, penetrating trauma to the pregnant patient most commonly injures the gravid uterus.[12] The use of peritoneal lavage is well accepted. Its contraindications do include the gravid patient especially late in gestation. Other contraindications include previous abdominal surgery, which may cause adhesions between hollow viscera and the anterior abdominal wall. The configuration of intra-abdominal anatomy may pose two hazards to diagnostic peritoneal lavage: 1) the technique may injure an adherent viscus, and 2) the resultant localization of fluid or blood may prevent its adequate aspiration and thus render the test falsely negative.

The trauma patient in her third trimester of pregnancy may still be evaluated for the presence of surgically significant intraabdominal pathology by peritoneal lavage if certain cautions are entertained.[13] The patient's bladder should be evacuated, either spontaneously or by urethral catheterization. The lavage site should be as far craniad as possible from the fundus of the uterus. Thus whereas peritoneal lavage is generally executed through an infraumbilical incision in the midline, the procedure should be carried out by way of a supraumbilical approach in the gravid patient, especially late in gestation. A number of techniques are available for the determination and include the direct surgical approach for insertion of a dialysis or similar catheter, the percutaneous intra peritoneal Seldinger technique, and insertion of a similar sized catheter. Either approach is acceptable, and the decision relates more to the personal experience of the physician than to the theoretical benefits of the technique. Approximately 1 L of crystalloid should be infused as rapidly as tolerated. After a brief period of time (minutes) and agitation as tolerated by the patient's abdomen, the infused fluid should be evacuated. The removal of approximately 750 mL of unfused fluid is probably the average aspirate after a peritoneal lavage with 1 L, and should suffice for diagnostic purposes. This test is 95% accurate according to most reviews and thus is highly specific for the presence of surgically signficant intraabdominal trauma. However one must respect the 5% false-negative–false-positive figure. Among these categories, the false-negative figure is about 2%. Thus, should doubt exist despite a "negative" peritoneal lavage, laparotomy should not be obviated.

The Levin tube (nasogastric) drainage may be clear despite through and through penetration of the stomach whether by pointed instrument or by missile. Although essential in the management of the trauma victim, this diagnostic and therapeutic tool has its limitations. The same is not true for a Foley (bladder) catheter. Rarely does penetrating trauma of the upper urinary tract fail to produce gross blood within the urinary tract, and hence such bleeding becomes evident in the bladder catheter drainage. This finding indicates intravenous pyelography and, if that proves negative, then cystography, but not cystoscopy for obvious reasons. When blunt trauma is causal, both intravenous pyelography and cystography are indicated since the likelihood of multiple injuries to the urinary tract is a consideration. Blood exiting the urethra is an indication for an attempt at gentle passage of a soft rubber catheter through the urethra and into the bladder. If such is not possible, the urethrography is indicated since urethral injury is implied. Although more common in men, the traumatic injury to the urethra of women is not rare and becomes a serious complication of pregnancy and trauma, since repair of the damaged urethra now becomes problematic. Should it be accomplished immediately after the injury, after the delivery, or as a later staged urethral reconstruction, assuming that urethral stricture is the ultimate outcome? Space does not permit discussion of all of these controversies, but suffice it to say that maternal welfare is the overriding criteria on her cause of shock must be addressed by whatever means to include any and all diagnostic indications and available facilities.

Use of the medical or military antishock trousers (MAST) has found wide implementation in the management of trauma victims, particularly those in hypovolemic shock. The pregnant patient is no exception, other than that as she approaches term the pressures delivered by the MAST must not be of such magnitude as to induce abortion or other obstetrical complications. Likewise, the physician or other allied health professional must ascertain that the urinary bladder is relatively empty either by history, by spontaneous voiding, or by urinary bladder catheterization; otherwise, the possibility of bladder rupture exists and may complicate the employment of the MAST. The latter autotransfuses approximately 2 units of whole blood. It applies pressure to the capacitance vessels of the lower extremities, pelvis and abdomen. The latter vessels along with those in the more craniad portion of the body are relatively large systemic veins that contain up to 60% of circulating blood volume. Obviously this blood is crossmatched and type specific. It is usually also sterile, and anticoagulation is unnecessary. With the above precautions in mind the MAST can be utilized in the field when shock is obvious, and successful therapy is dependent upon whole blood infusion and surgical correction of the source of bleeding. Whether to risk fetal death secondary to maternal (and fetal) systemic arterial hypotension from failure to institute the autotransfusion subsequent to inflation of the MAST or to risk spontaneous or induced abortion by inflation of the garment is a judgmental call. Few have sufficient experience to pontificate on such decisions.

Once inflated, the MAST must be carefully monitored. Changes in altitude and temperature significantly influence the pressure generated by the garment upon the lower body. Thus, if the victim is transported from a cold environment (such as the street) to a warm environment (such as the transporting vehicle or the treatment facility), those responsible for the patient's care must be cognizant of the fact that the change in temperature and its increase will augment the pressure within the garment. Too great a pressure is thereby a potential hazard. Most MAST have built-in pressure excess devices to prevent the excess buildup of defined forces. But the tolerance of these "escape valves" approaches 90 mmHg and such a valve would be poorly tolerated by the gravid woman, probably regardless of gestational duration. A change in altitude will have similar problematic considerations. Should aeromedical evacuation of a pregnant casualty be required, it must be recognized that in an unpressurized vehicle, such as a helicopter, altitude will reduce external pressure upon the MAST thus increasing the force it delivers to the patient. Obviously the reverse holds true during descent to the treating facility. Appreciation of these fundamentals should enhance the successful utilization of the MAST in the trauma victim who is pregnant. Additional consideration in the preoperative management of the hypotensive pregnant trauma victim include those physiologic phenomena that accompany pregnancy particularly as term approaches. Several additional considerations are pertinent to the preoperative management of the obstetrical victim of trauma who is in shock. Near term hypovolemia is characteristic and becomes a two-edged sword. Although this phenomenon may protect the mother in her response to shock the same is not true for her fetus, who tolerates hypotension much less well. Thus, the MAST must not be deflated until provision is made for several units of blood for simultaneous infusion when deflation is indicated.

Leukocytosis (up to 20,000 leukocytes per mm^3) is common near term. This factor plays a role in the assessment of the victim of traumatic shock who is also pregnant. Rarely does septic shock complicate the pregnant victim of trauma to a degree that requires alteration of the basic resuscitation measures already described. However, the knowledge that leukocytosis is a frequent accompaniment of pregnancy should alert the treating physician to the fact that the leukocyte count may be a false indicator of the magnitude of the problem. It may be elevated above normal levels (5000 to 10,000 leukocytes) which is consistent with near term pregnancy. However, septic shock may be characterized by leukopenia which in the near-term patient may be relative in terms of absolute numbers. Rarely is septic shock a consideration for the physician treating the pregnant patient who is a victim of trauma. Nonetheless, this must be considered as a diagnostic alternative to the cause for hypotension in the gravid woman who has been a victim of trauma. Recall that septic shock is frequently accompanied by leukopenia and thus the relative leukocytosis of pregnancy becomes more problematic in terms of implications of abnormally high or low levels of the count. The pregnant patient near term has a relative venous hypotension.

This factor is of important concern to the treating physician, whose attempts at circulatory blood volume replacement may prove to be problematic. In addition, near term implies a larger uterus whose position may compromise venous return to the right heart by physical interruption of blood flow through the vena cava.[14] Thus every effort should be made to position the near term gravid trauma patient on her left side. Alternative positions such as the recumbent or, worse yet, the right lateral decubitus position aggravate the already existing hypotension by interrupting blood flow to the heart. Often procedural requirements preclude optimal positioning of the patient, but whenever possible these considerations deserve attention.

Additionally, the pregnant trauma victim near term will exhibit a degree of hydronephrosis and hydroureter which would otherwise be considered abnormal, but which in pregnancy is not abnormal and relates to the fact that the enlarging uterus distributes direct pressure upon the ureters as they cross the brim of the pelvis.[15] Thus, radiographic identification (IVP) of these findings may be consistent with gestation particularly near term and may not necessarily be construed as abnormal.

Should surgery be required to constrain life-threatening hemorrhage numerous considerations are pertinent to the management of the gravid victim of trauma. Her health and well-being have been addressed. The patient and the family must be consulted as to the threat of life of both mother and fetus. Hopefully, a decision commmensurate with the patient's successful outcome will be determined. We would favor a midline laparotomy for the more common indications for surgical intervention in the pregnant trauma victim. Whether the trauma is blunt or penetrating, the likelihood of injury to the spleen or small bowel is problematic when trauma to the pregnant patient occurs. Shock must be addressed with rapidity. Often surgery is the only recourse. Through a midline incision extending from xyphoid to pubis all of the intraabdominal organs can be addressed and the appropriate treatment instituted. Numerous considerations participate in decision making at this point.

Fetal monitoring, especially via ultrasonography where feasible, has been instituted, and presumably the fetus is still viable. If not, surgery is contraindicated with a few rare exceptions which include sudden cessation of fetal heart sounds and sudden evidence of fetal demise based upon evaluation of this parameter. Where doubt exists, however, surgery is indicated since little morbidity and negligible mortality should attend laparotomy even in the gravid patient. Once the need for laparotomy or even thoracotomy is determined, haste should be exercised in attempts to control life (lives)-threatening hypotension. The operating surgeon must recognize that hypotension is the greatest threat to fetal survival in the wake of trauma to the mother.

Operative control of shock is not germane to this chapter, but remains a concern regarding preoperative management. There are indications for hysterectomy as well as caesarean section when trauma complicates pregnancy. These must be discussed with the family and the patient whenever possible. Important considerations regarding the mother must take precedence over the decision of the operating surgeon with regard to the welfare of both mother and fetus. If the fetus is dead as determined by most criteria, then the surgeon's choice of action is less problematic. Threat to life from exsanguination is of high priority and must be addressed rapidly. Likewise, should shock accompany maternal injury when term is near, then caesarean section is appropriate to save both mother and fetus. Should maternal hypovolemia and shock be the result of major vessel injury, then hysterectomy may be required for the exposure necessary to control hemorrhage from major vessels such as the aorta or the inferior vena cava. Should injury to the fetus, its umbilical cord, or placenta be suspect, then again surgery to control injury and attendant shock is indicated. The decision as to what procedure should be carried out remains with the operating surgeon. Should the fetus be defined as dead, then attention should be directed towards maternal survival. Occasionally, the fetus is identified as dead or, worse yet, infected. When these conditions accompany trauma to a gravid patient the surgical choices become more applicable to the mother than to her fetus. Rapid evacuation of the conceptus and control of hemorrhage is indicated. The use of broad-spectrum antibiotics is also indicated. Not to be minimized is the need to address tetanus immunizational status. Most service men and women have been, by definition, immunized against tetanus. The history is sufficient for decision making, but when lacking, then immunization by tetanus toxoid as well as human immune globulin is indicated.

The choice of anesthetic agent, should surgery be necessary, is controversial. Threats to the fetus as well as to the mother are considered. Often the need for prompt control of hemorrhage precludes appropriate assessment. This problem is addressed in Chapter 4 in detail. Appropriate corrective measures are indicated and essential to the outcome of both.[16] Recall that maternal welfare correlates fetal survival when the two are victims of trauma. Thus, a Catholic approach to the victim of trauma who is pregnant is scientifically as well as ethically appropriate. All too frequently, the fate of the conceptus is given higher priority than that of the mother. The success of pregnancy is dependent upon maternal welfare. Should the mother sustain shock for an unwarranted period of time then the likelihood of a successful pregnancy will become problematic regardless of the source of trauma.

REFERENCES

1. Report of the National Center for Health Statistics, September 1981.
2. *ACS Advanced Trauma Life Support Syllabus.* Chicago, Ill,

American College of Surgeons, 1982.

3. Swan KG: *Trauma Management—Historical Perspectives Clinical Update*, vol 1. Princeton, NJ, Nassau Publications, 1982, p 1.
4. Swan KG, Swan RC Jr: *Gunshot Wounds*. Littleton, MA, PSG Publishing Co. Inc, 1980.
5. Renser M, Ven De Putte I, Vermylen C: Massive fetomaternal hemorrhage as a cause of perinatal mortality and morbidity. *Europ J Obstet Gynecol Reprod Biol*, 1976;6:125.
6. Shahar E, Birenbaum E, Inbar D, et al: Hypovolemic shock at birth due to extensive fetomaternal hemorrhage. *I J Med Sci* 1981;17:441.
7. Hedberg E, Radberg C, Sannun R: Radiological pelvimetry in cases of intra-uterine asphyxia. *Acta Obstet Gynecol Scand* 1968;47:87.
8. Prichard JA, MacDonald PC: *William's Obstetrics*, ed 16. New York, Appleton Century Crofts, 1980.
9. Pepperell RJ, Rubinstein E, MacIssac IA: Motor-car accidents during pregnancy. *Med J Aust* 1977;1:203,659.
10. Crosby WM: Automotive trauma and the pregnant patient. *Contemporary Ob/Gyn* 1976;8:115.
11. Lowe RJ, Saletta JD, Read DR, et al: Should laparotomy be mandatory or selective in gunshot wounds of the abdomen? *J Trauma* 1977;17:903.
12. Rothenberger D, Quattlebaum FW, Perry JF Jr, et al: Blunt maternal trauma: A review of 103 cases. *J Trauma* 1978;18:173.
13. Haycock CE: Saving both the mother and fetus. *Consultant* 1982;269.
14. Buschbaum HJ: Traumatic injury in pregnancy in Barber HRK, Graber EA (eds): *Surgical Diseases in Pregnancy*. Philadelphia, The WB Saunders Co, 1974, Chapter 12.
15. Greenhill JP: *Obstetrics*, ed 13. Philadelphia, The WB Saunders Co, 1965.
16. Baker DP: Trauma in the pregnant patient. *Surg Clin North Am* 1982;2:275.

CHAPTER 4

BLUNT TRAUMA IN PREGNANCY

CHRISTINE E. HAYCOCK

Although there are increasing numbers of victims of penetrating trauma encountered in the United States because of inner city violence involving knives and guns, as mentioned in an earlier chapter, blunt traumas caused by vehicular accidents, falls from heights, and blows from blunt weapons, fists, and feet still lead the injury list. Automobiles generally are the major cause of injury.[1-10]

The key to the treatment of such patients is accurate diagnosis of the specific injury involved or at least recognition that an injury requiring immediate attention or at least close observation is present. This is especially true when dealing with the pregnant patient where two lives may well be at stake, that of the mother and her developing fetus.

Earlier chapters have discussed the physiologic and anatomical changes of pregnancy, so they will not be reiterated here except as relevant to the discussion. Diagnostic methodology is well covered in Chapter 3 so that repetition here will again be minimal.

Blunt trauma to the abdomen most commonly results in injury to the solid organs: spleen, liver, kidneys, and pancreas. The mobility of most areas of the gastrointestinal tract minimize injury to these structures except at fixed points such as the duodenum, cecum, hepatic and splenic flexures of the colon and the anorectal area.

The enlarging uterus might seem a very vulnerable target for blunt trauma, but it is a markedly resilient organ and can sustain quite severe pressure without rupture. This does not mean, however, that the developing fetus within the uterus may not sustain injury despite the buffering action of the amniotic fluid.

Stuart and colleagues from the Department of Obstetrics at Western Ontario University in Canada reported two cases of fetal death in 1980 after what appeared to be minor blunt trauma to the mother.[11] In both cases, because the mother appeared to be stable, delay occurred in diagnosing injury to the fetus. It was not until the fetal hearts were not heard with a fetoscope and their absence was confirmed by doppler ultrasonography and the presence of a small amount of bright red vaginal bleeding that the injuries were recognized, and then it was too late. Vaginal bleeding after abdominal trauma to the pregnant woman is always an ominous sign relative to the pregnancy since it often is indicative of placental separation.[12]

The first patient had been wearing an improperly placed seat belt; the second, who was not wearing a seat belt, was crushed against the steering wheel of the car.

This brings up two important points regarding the use of seat belts in automobiles by pregnant patients: 1) they should be worn, and 2) they must be worn properly.

Matthews noted that Australia has a mandatory seat belt regulation which means that the belt must be worn whether or not the wearer is pregnant.[13] He reported a case of a 23-week pregnant woman wearing a very loosely fitted lap-shoulder harness when involved in a head-on collision. As a result, the lap belt caused a rupture of the uterus with an 8-cm tear across the anterior fundus, leaving the fetus and placenta lying loose in the abdominal cavity. Fortunately, with good emergency resuscitation the uterus was repaired and the mother was saved, although the fetus was lost.

Crosby and Costiloe studied 208 cases of pregnant victims of severe automobile accidents in the United States. Of these cases, 28 patients wore seat belts; as a result, maternal death was reduced from 7.8% to 3.6%, but with a nonstatistically significant increase in fetal loss from 14.4% to 16.7%.[14]

These authors studied the forces directed against the uterus as the mother was jack-knifed forward over the lap belt (no shoulder belt was worn). The abdomen and uterus flex over the restraining belt, which elevates intrauterine pressure and distorts the size and shape of the uterus. This can cause placental detachment (the most common cause of fetal death in blunt trauma) by a shearing action.

Matthews, however, points out that actual rupture of the uterus usually only occurs when the lap belt is too loosely fastened and slides up over the uterus, applying direct force to the fundus, and hence it ruptures.[13]

The addition of the shoulder harness or belt, again when properly worn, can also aid in prevention of injury to the uterus and fetus by preventing the jack-knifing described by Crosby and Costiloe.

Physicians are advised to caution their pregnant patients to wear seat lap and shoulder belts to save their own lives in automobile collisions, but to wear them properly fastened to protect the developing fetus.

The lap belt should be worn snug and low over the pelvis, and the shoulder belt should be directed to the side of the abdomen (Figure 4-1). The best type of harness would, of course, be the double shoulder strap type worn by race drivers, but since that is not practical, the lap-shoulder type with the buckle on the side is the safest for the pregnant patient.[15] This was also pointed out by McCormick, who reported a case of traumatic rupture of the uterus by an improperly worn seat belt.[16]

In addition to the injuries to the uterus, improperly (and occasionally even properly) worn belts have been responsible for injuries ranging from the rupture of solid and hollow viscera and diaphragmatic rupture to decapitation.[17–19]

Look for a telltale mark across the abdominal wall, usually a narrow, erythematous contusion matching the width of the

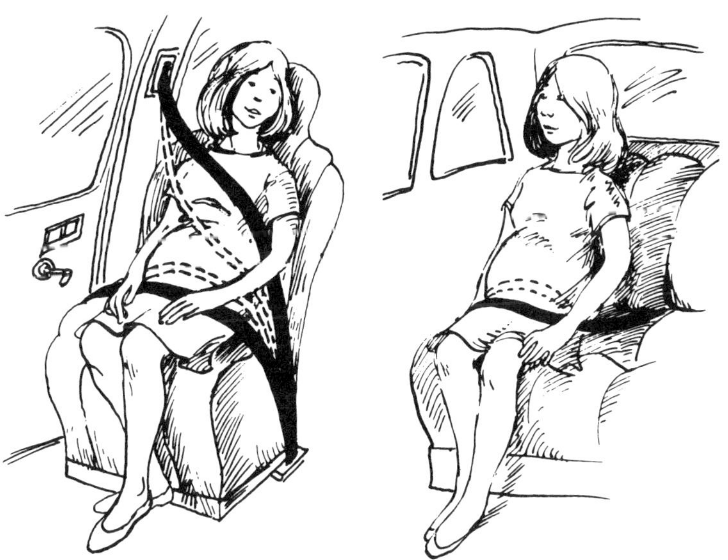

Figure 4-1 Dotted lines indicate improper placement of seat belts. Solid lines show correct placement. Reproduced by permission of *Consultant Magazine.*

belt. If it is present, assume intraabdominal injury until absolutely proven otherwise.

In a 12-year study conducted by Elliott in 1966 in Brisbane, Australia, of traffic accidents involving 39 pregnant patients, fatal injuries were sustained by eight women. Although most of them had multiple injuries, death was primarily due to severe hemorrhage, either intraabdominal or retroperitoneal.[20]

Better emergency care with the ability we now have to replace fluid volume more rapidly might well have saved some of these patients. Such a typical case was reported by Punnonen of Finland in 1974.[21]

When the mother's death has occurred, it does not always mean that the life of the fetus has been lost. The *American Medical Association News* in 1983 reported the birth of a healthy baby born to a legally dead woman 64 days after brain death had been established.[22] Similar cases were reported by Sampson and Peterson in 1977[23] and by Lucas in 1976.[24] In this latter case the mother ultimately also survived her coma.

A more spectacular case occurred in Quincy, IL, in 1971.[25] A 30-year-old near-term woman was driving her car when she lost control and it went off the highway. She was thrown out of the car as it traveled some 525 feet off the road. When people arrived on the scene they heard an infant crying. An alive, uninjured, 8-lb, 10 oz baby girl was found some 400 feet off the highway. The mother was dead. She had sustained an evisceration of the abdomen with a laceration of the fundus of the uterus delivering the infant. The chances are that the amniotic sac protected the infant as it bounced on to the ground and then burst open delivering the infant.

Other authors have reported successful postmortem caesarean sections with infant survival.[26] This points up the fact that one should never give up on the survival of the fetus until every effort has been made to establish its viability.

Dr. Cohen-Addad in Chapter 10 will cover the types of injuries usually sustained by the fetus in blunt trauma; however, it can be noted that the most common injuries are fractures of the skull, clavicles, and the upper extremities, probably due to the normal upright position of the fetus in the uterus. Fractures of the pelvis and lower extremities do occur, but are relatively rare.

It was mentioned earlier that premature separation of the placenta can occur not infrequently in severe blunt trauma. The number of such cases reported in the literature points up the need to reiterate the vital necessity of careful fetal monitoring all throughout the resuscitative efforts for the injured mother.[27–29] The need to document these findings to protect the physician from later legal consequences is detailed in articles by Eaton and Danziger[30] and in the *British Medical Journal*.[31] Continuous monitoring should persist for at least 24 hours. The advent of real time ultrasonography augmented by computerized tomography scans has reduced the patient's exposure to x-ray irradiation as well as enhanced the trauma surgeon and obstetrician's ability to monitor their patients (mother and fetus). Lacking these sophisticated devices, however, the simple use of the fetoscope by a well trained nurse constantly listening for fetal heart sounds in the emergency department can be invaluable to the surgeon who must decide when and whether to operate on the blunt traumatized pregnant patient.

Some physicians have questioned the use of peritoneal lavage in the pregnant patient for fear of puncture of the uterus or intestines. However, when the establishment of the rapid diagnosis of intraabdominal hemorrhage is required, the procedure can be safely carried out above the umbilicus if the uterus is at or above the umbilicus by using the same precautions as in the non-pregnant patient, ie, emptying the bladder and avoiding abdominal scars from previous surgery. If severe shock is present the procedure is unnecessary, as the diagnosis should be obvious.

Although automobile accidents cause the majority of blunt trauma to pregnant women, falls, kicks, and blows do also account for such injuries. Less frequently, however, do these types of blows cause fetal injury.[32] It is not uncommon for fractures to occur to the fetus that may go unnoticed (eg, a women beaten by her husband may not report for treatment) until at delivery the injury is found. A minor fall might also result in fetal injury, especially fracture, if the patient falls directly forward on her abdomen.

If the injury to the mother is not sufficient to require laparotomy, but ultrasonography after the loss of heart sounds has confirmed fetal death, this does not mean that caesarean section is necessary or required. If a spontaneous delivery does not occur immediately, there is no haste to introduce labor unless a coagulopathy (disseminated intravascular clotting) develops.[33] If uterine inertia prevents progression of labor once it has begun, or labor cannot be induced in the face of deteriorating vital signs in the mother, then caesarean section will be necessary.

Once a decision has been made to take the patient to surgery for operative intervention, there are a few comments that should be made in this regard.

Positioning of the patient on the table supine may lead to vena caval compression, so she should be brought to the operating room and placed initially during induction of anesthesia in the lateral position if at all possible. Once anesthesia is accomplished she can then be turned to the supine position. This will minimize the problem. It may also be feasible to tilt the table laterally during surgery.

Exploration should be carried out with a midline incision in the same manner as for the nonpregnant patient. Since good exposure to examine all organs is vital, the incision may have to extend from pubis to sternum. The uterus can be gently manuevered and displaced forward if required to examine the retroperitoneal area. Gentle handling of the uterus has not been shown to induce abortion, and the possibility of missing an injury outweighs this outcome in any event.

The examination of the abdomen is generally carried out in the same routine fashion as with any other trauma patient. One area, however, that deserves special mention is the diaphragm. Since any increasing intraabdominal pressure including pregnancy itself can produce a hiatal hernia, a special point should be made to check this area for an enlarged hiatus or diaphragmatic tear which can be overlooked and result in a problem that may surface much later. Such a case was presented by Dudley, et al in 1979.[34]

If fetal distress has been documented and caesarean section is planned, bleeding of any consequence from any other source such as the spleen or a large vessel must be dealt with first. Removal of the fetus with subsequent reduction in the size of the uterus may then facilitate additional exploration of the abdomen. Occasionally, the need for exposure may require emptying the uterus regardless of the survivability of the fetus.

Even though the the physician is in the abdominal cavity, if there is no fetal distress or injury to the uterus, it is not normally advised that caesarean section be done unless the patient is close to delivery. There is no point in bringing out a premature infant when there is a good possibility of continuation of the pregnancy to term. This is, however, a decision which must be made by the surgeon, neonatologist, and obstetrician working together in the best interests of the mother and fetus.

Closure of the abdomen with the uterus intact and large generally poses no problem. Retention sutures are generally advisable, however. Labor and delivery are generally tolerated well even within hours or days after laparotomy and in the presence of pelvic fractures.[35]

Thus, it is obvious that blunt trauma to the pregnant patient does entail certain special considerations not seen in the nonpregnant patient.

REFERENCES

1. Lane JC: Motor car accidents during pregnancy—I. *Med J Aust* 1977;1:669.
2. Ojwang SOB, Bennun M, Musila S: Uterine rupture due to road traffic accident. *East African Med J* 1978;55:14.
3. Handel CK: Case report of uterine rupture after an automobile accident. *J Reprod Med* 1978;20:90.
4. Connor E, Curran J: In utero traumatic intraabdominal deceleration injury to the fetus a case report. *Am J Obstet Gynecol* 1976; 125:567.
5. Golan A, Sandbana O, Teare AJ: Trauma in late pregnancy. A report of 15 cases. *S African Med J* 1980;57:161.
6. Weinstein EC, Pallias V: Rupture of the pregnant uterus from blunt trauma. *J Trauma* 1968;8:1111.
7. Galle PC, Anderson SG: A case of automobile trauma during pregnancy. *Obstet Gynecol* 1979;54:467.
8. Baijal E: Multiple fractures of the pelvis with an unusually wide disruption of the symphysis pubis sustained in an accident shortly after childbirth: A case report. *Injury* 1974;6:57.
9. Kalstone CE, Laros RK: Traumatic rupture of the non-pregnant uterus. *JAMA* 1969;208:2338.
10. Pepperell RJ, Rubinstein E, MacIsaac IA: Motor car accidents during pregnancy. *Obstet Gynecol* 1977;32:659.

11. Stuart GCE, Harding PGR, Davies EM: Blunt abdominal trauma in pregnancy. *Can Med Assoc J* 1980;122:901.
12. Heitzman ER, Markarian B: Vaginal bleeding after trauma in pregnant women. *N Y State J Med* 1970;70:2338.
13. Matthews CD: Incorrectly used seat belt associated with uterine rupture following vehicular collision. *Am J Obstet Gynecol* 1975; 121:1115.
14. Crosby WM, Costiloe JP: Safety of lap-belt restraint for pregnant victims of automobile collisions. *N Engl J Med* 1971;284:632.
15. Haycock CE: Injury during pregnancy: Saving both mother and fetus. *Consultant* 1982;22:269.
16. McCormick RD: Seat belt injury: Case of complete transection of pregnant uterus. *JAOA* 1968;67:1139.
17. Poulson AM, Gabert HA: Fetal death secondary to nonpenetrating trauma to the gravid uterus. *Am J Obstet Gynecol* 1973;116:580.
18. Ericcson CD: Lap-belt restraints in pregnancy. *N Engl J Med* 1971; 284:1271.
19. Whitehouse DB: Hazard to fetus from safety harness. *Br Med J* 1972;798:510.
20. Elliott M: Vehicular accidents and pregnancy. *Aust New Eng J Obstet Gynecol* 1966;6:279.
21. Punnonen R: Traumatic premature separation of placenta: Report of a case. *Ann Chir Gynaecol Fenn* 1974;63:487.
22. Healthy baby born to legally dead woman. *American Medical Association News* 15 April 1973, p 19.
23. Sampson MB, Peterson LP: Post-traumatic coma during pregnancy. *Obstet Gynecol* 1979;53:2S.
24. Lucas B: Nursing care study: Pregnant car-crash victim. *Nurse Times* 1976; 72:451.
25. Griep EA: Traumatic live birth of normal infant. *JAMA* 1971; 217:477.
26. Smith GE: Postmortem caesarean section. A case report. *J Obstet Gynaecol Br Commonw* 1973;80:181.
27. Powell HDW: Accidental pelvic disruption in pregnancy with other injuries. *Proc Royal Soc Med* 1966;59:706.
28. Crosby WM: Trauma during pregnancy: Maternal and fetal injury. *Obstet Gynecol Surg* 1974;29:683.
29. Peyser MR, Toaff R: Traumatic rupture of the placenta. A rare case of fetal death. *Obstet Gynecol* 1969;34:561.
30. Eaton CJ, Danziger RF: Traumatic disruption of pregnancy. Report of a case and its legal implications. *Obstet Gynecol* 1967;30:16.
31. Right of fetus to sue. *Br Med J* 1973;847:244.
32. Fort AT, Harlin RS: Pregnancy outcome after noncatastrophic

maternal trauma during pregnancy. *Obstet Gynecol* 1970;35:912.

33. Marx GF, Steen SN, Arkins RE, et al: Coagulopathy in pregnant woman following car accident. *N Y State J Med* 1969;69:1196.
34. Dudley AG, Teaford H, Gatewood TS Jr: Delayed traumatic rupture of the diaphragm in pregnancy. *Obstet Gynecol* 1979;53:25S.
35. Speer DP, Peltier LF: Pelvic fractures and pregnancy. *J Trauma* 1972;12:474.

CHAPTER 5

PENETRATING TRAUMA IN PREGNANCY

CHRISTINE E. HAYCOCK

Unlike blunt trauma, penetrating injuries can cause uterine injuries to the patient during any stage of pregnancy. The bony pelvis is little protection against a high velocity bullet. Penetrating wounds are more likely than blunt trauma to cause multiple abdominal organ injury unless the blunt trauma is very severe. The larger the uterus, the more apt it is to be injured.

Stab wounds with knives, ice picks, and even pitchforks have been reported. Iatrogenic injuries involving some recent invasive genetic studies are also beginning to appear in the literature, but are not as yet well documented.[1]

Stab wounds have amazingly not proved to be a major source of uterine injury despite the frequency with which this type of lesion is seen in the emergency departments of our inner cities. Although stab wounds can have devastating results, it is also true that a knife can be thrust into the abdomen and pulled out without any important injury. The omentum may be the only structure injured, and it has usually stopped bleeding when the abdomen is opened.

It was the rule at most university hospitals that all stab wounds as well as gunshot wounds of the abdomen must be explored. This is now mainly true only for gunshot wounds, as discussed below.

Peritoneal lavage has proven to be 94% to 96% accurate in diagnosing damage from blunt abdominal trauma, although it is somewhat less accurate when applied to stab wounds since penetration of the intestines may occur that does not immediately give a positive lavage, but only becomes obvious when peritoneal irritation due to sepsis develops.[2] Some authors have advocated careful serial observation of such patients as an acceptable alternative to lavage, although most also use lavage when in real doubt.[3,4] Other modalities include laparoscopy or peritoneoscopy which can be performed best in the operating room just before celiotomy if the diagnosis remains in doubt. This procedure, however, would be difficult in the third trimester of pregnancy. These results have also been reported as about 96% accurate.[5,6]

Jordan has described the ultraconservative management of trauma in general.[7] However, when the life of the fetus is also at stake, conservatism, which might allow better stabilization of the mother to insure the survival of the fetus, is not without its merits. Laparotomies that ultimately are negative may pose a risk in this regard.

Even when the knife blade has penetrated the uterus it does not always mean the loss of the fetus. Survival of the fetus after repair of knife caused perforations of the uterus has been reported in the literature and seen at the University Hospital in Newark.

Badia and Charleton,[8] Wright et al[9] and Jordan[10] have all reported cases where fetal survival has followed the repair of a uterine perforation. In these cases the fetus was not injured. In a case reported by McNabney and Smith the fetus was injured and after delivery, also had to be explored. Fortunately, both mother and infant survived.[11] Results reported by Moss et al[12] and Dyer and Barclay[13] were not as fortunate, as the fetal injuries resulted in death. In one case death was due to severing of the umbilical cord by the weapon.

The reason for the much higher rate of survival from stab wounds as opposed to gunshot wounds lies in the mechanism of injury. Stab wounds generally confine the area of injury to the track of the weapon as it enters and exits. If the knife is twisted, or the wound is made by a slash with a weapon such as a machete, damage may be extensive, but still is confined to the paths of the blade. Hence, the area of injury can often be predicted.

A review of 469 stab wounds at the University Hospital in Newark, NJ from 1972 to 1975 revealed that the left upper quadrant was the target in 146 cases, and the right upper quadrant was the target in 99 cases (Table 5-1). Of these same cases the liver and small bowel were the most frequently injured (these were nonpregnant women and men). Only one patient of 46 women suffered injury to the reproductive organs, and that was an ovary (Table 5-2). This in part would explain the low injury rate even to the uterus in pregnant women.

Gunshot wounds are not as predictable and, in fact, may strike any portion of the abdomen or the body resulting in serious injury that can directly or indirectly affect the outcome of a pregnancy. Exploration remains mandatory for all abdominal gunshot wounds as confirmed by a study by Lowe in 1977.[14]

Survival of the fetus such as that reported by Browns et al in 1977, is rare, especially when a gunshot wound penetrates the abdomen and strikes the fetus.[15] In his case the bullet lodged in

Table 5-1
Location of Wounds Described

	No. of Wounds
Left upper quadrant	146
Right upper quadrant	99
Epigastric	75
Left flank	31
Left lower quadrant	30
Right lower quadrant	26
Right flank	23
Back	21
Lower midline	12
Pelvic	6

Table 5-2
Structures Injured

Organ	No. of Wounds	Organ	No. of Wounds
Liver	122	Diaphragm	33
Small bowel	108	Kidney	30
Major vessels	67	Pancreas	26
Spleen	58	Bladder	14
Colon	58	Gall Bladder	12
Omentum	54	Ureter	7
Stomach	41	Appendix	2
Mesentery	33	Ovary	1
		Adrenal	1

the fetus's upper arm after traversing the abdomen from an entrance in the posterior flank and exiting the right anterior chest. The infant was delivered by caesarean section after it was ascertained that only the uterus was injured. Subsequently, laparotomy was done on the infant, and repair of its injuries was successfully carried out.

As Browns correctly pointed out, fetal mortality after wounding is high whereas maternal morbidity is low. This is due to the protection afforded the mother by absorption of the kinetic energy of the missile by the uterus protecting her frequently from further injury. Fetal survival depends on how close the fetus is to term, since a near-term infant can withstand caesarean section and celiotomy if required, whereas a premature infant cannot.

Another interesting survival of a fetus was reported in 1976 by Gysler et al in Switzerland.[16] Both mother and infant in this case were seriously injured. The mother sustained damage to her intestines and uterus and the infant had a bullet lodged in its thymus gland. After a caesarean section was done both survived exploratory surgery.

The majority of earlier cases, however, have not been as fortunate. Buchsbaum in 1975 reported on a collected series of 70 cases of wounds to the uterus with a 66% perinatal mortality.[17]

For those surgeons who may not be familiar with the mechanism of injury in gunshot wounds it might be well to review these so that a better understanding of the reasons for the severity of these wounds is obtained. Surgeons who deal frequently with such cases tend to overlook the fact that their colleagues in less turbulent area hospitals may seldom encounter such injuries.

The difficulty with gunshot wounds is that the area of injury is not confined to the tract of the bullet, but extends at right angles due to the kinetic energy dissipated by the missile. This kinetic energy is measured by the formula:

$$KE = (M \times V^2)/2,$$

where M is the weight of the bullet in grains, V is the velocity in feet per second squared, and the arbitrary factor for gravity is 2. This formulation is simplified by the Swan brothers in their book, *Gunshot Wounds*. They state that the kinetic energy is proportional ($KE \sim MV^2$) to the mass of the missile.[18]

This measured kinetic energy is present at the muzzle of the weapon. The further the bullet travels, the wind velocity, rain, or what it passes through – a door, a book, clothing – all slow the velocity to some degree. The striking energy is the kinetic energy that remains as the missile strikes the target. If the missile passes through the body it takes some residual energy with it. If it remains within the body all of its energy is imparted to the target organs.

Doubling the mass of the bullet may make a larger entrance wound, but since doubling the velocity quadruples the energy factor, the velocity is of more importance than the size of the missile is so far as tissue damage is concerned. Thus, for example, a high powered rifle with a muzzle velocity of 2800 feet per second will obviously cause more damage than a 38-caliber police weapon with a muzzle velocity of 850 feet per second.

In addition to the mass and velocity factors, the missile may also be tumbling end over end or deviating from its axis in the line of flight (yawing) and may thus strike the body sidewise rather than point on, often fragmenting first, thus inflicting more damage.

Shotguns are particularly devastating at close range because there are multiple missiles striking in a close pattern. Further away they spread out and, since the individual pellet's velocity is usually low they may only penetrate the skin and subcutaneous tissues. This is, however, dependent on the type of shell used, the size of the pellets, and the amount of powder. It is unnecessary to go into details in this regard for the scope of this discussion.

As the missile strikes the body the kinetic energy is dissipated along the tract of the bullet. Thus, the tissue damage generally extends beyond what is seen by the naked eye, necessitating sufficient debridement to ensure that all damaged tissue is removed.

There is also a cavitation effect especially evident with high-velocity missiles as the kinetic energy actually pushes tissues away from the path of the bullet creating a transient cavity around it that collapses and expands (reverberates) and may act as a vacuum to pull in such things as dirt, pieces of clothing, etc (Figures 5-1 and 5-2). Thus, bone may be broken or ligaments and vessels may be torn even though the bullet itself never touches them.

Fortunately, most civilian injuries occur as the result of low velocity handgun missiles so that this cavitation effect is minimal. Organs such as the liver and spleen are also more easily damaged in this fashion than are elastic tissues such as lung or muscle. If the bullet fragments, the pieces may each act as an individual missile, thus resulting in multiple injury tracts.

Wilson and Swartz in their review of wounds of the gravid uterus in 1972[19] included a number of cases of grenade, bomb or shrapnel injuries to this structure, and in areas of the world where conflicts still rage, such wounds must be relatively common, if not reported, as civilian populations comes under fire (Figures 5-3, 5-4, 5-5, and 5-6).

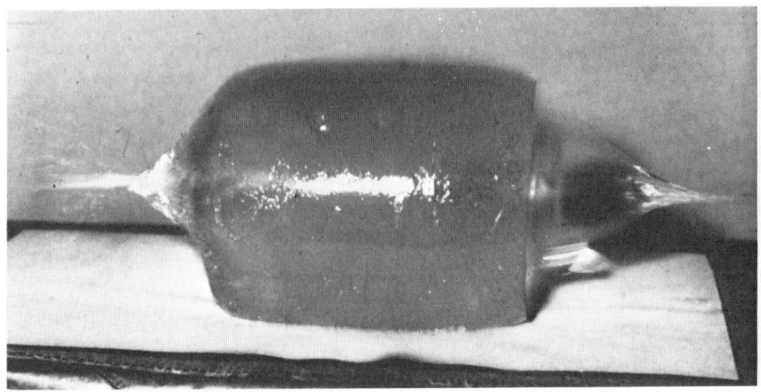

Figure 5-1 A 22-caliber rifle bullet is shown passing through a cylinder of gelatin from right to left. A glass rod placed below the path of the bullet is fractured due to lateral kinetic force, not by being struck by the missile.

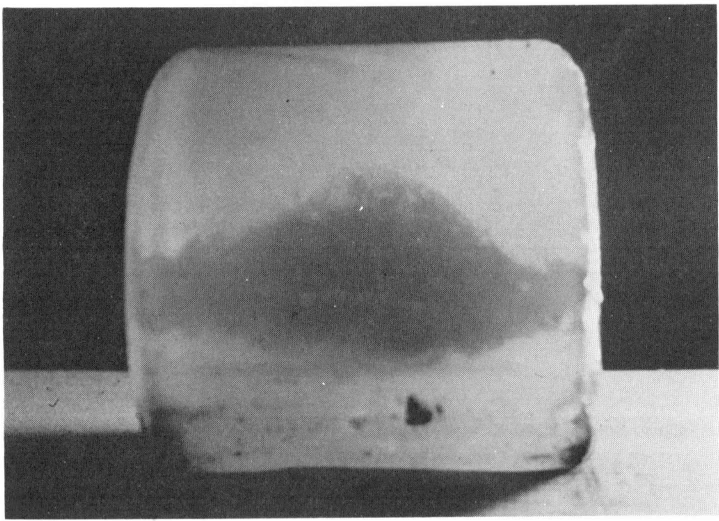

Figure 5-2 After the bullet has passed through the gelatin block, the extent of the injured area is made apparent by the use of dye. The cavitation effect is evident.

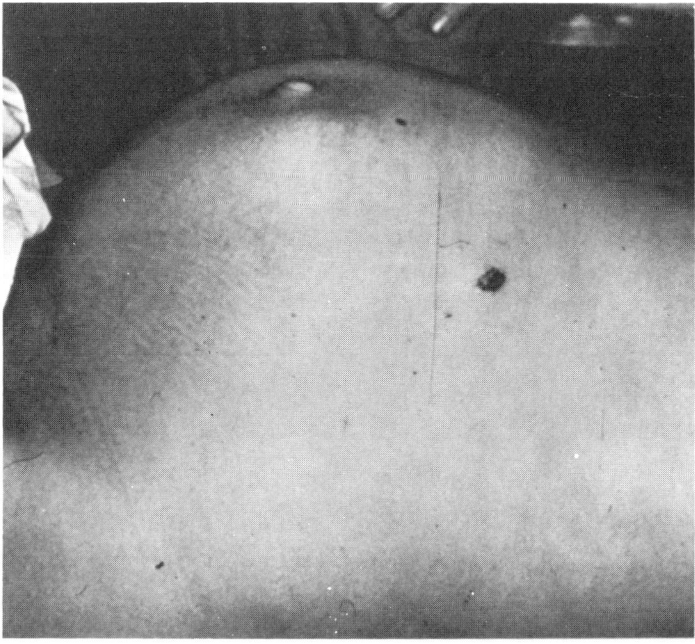

Figure 5-3 An M-2 carbine missile wound of the abdomen of a 23-year-old civilian in Vietnam, 7 months pregnant. Reproduced with permission from Swan KG, Swan RG: *Gunshot Wounds.* Littleton, MA, PSG Publishing Co, Inc, 1980.

More typical are cases such as the one reported by Wray and Burnett in 1971.[20] A pregnant patient sustained a low-velocity gunshot wound to the abdomen which resulted in injuries to the small intestines, uterus, and placenta. Celiotomy was done, and a caesarean section was performed. Although the infant initially was unresponsive, successful resuscitation was accomplished. The bullet had penetrated through the uterus from the right to left posterior aspects at its midportion, lacerating the placenta. The uterus was evacuated, the holes in

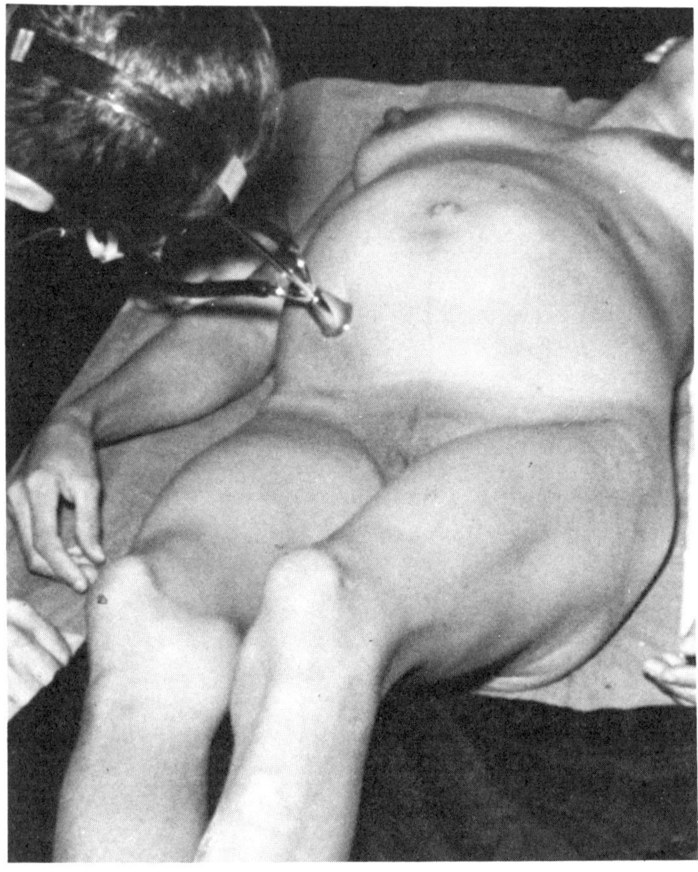

Figure 5-4 Immediate auscultation of the abdomen for fetal heart sounds in the same patient. The fetus was viable. Photo courtesy of Kenneth G. Swan, MD.

the uterus and intestines were repaired, and the patient made an uneventful recovery. Two years later, she had a second child delivered by caesarean section without difficulty.

Other such cases have been reported by Buchsbaum and Caruso[21] and Farzanfar and Shell.[22] An unusual case of criminal

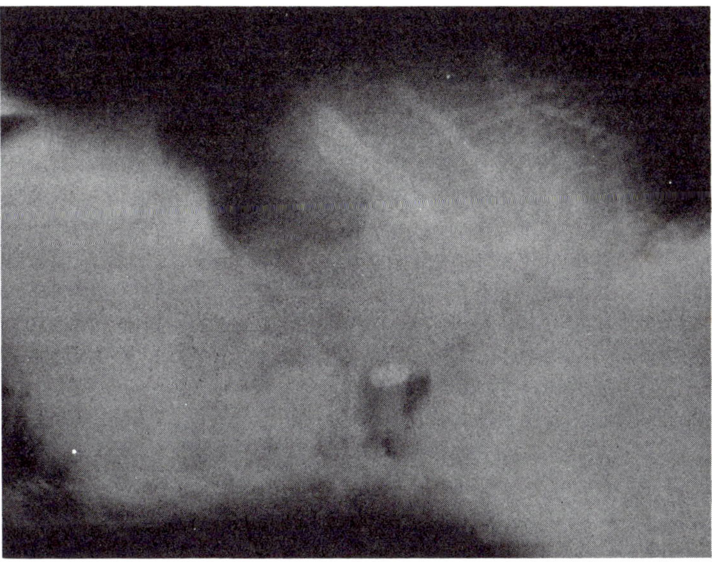

Figure 5-5 X-ray of the abdomen showing the bullet in place and fetal parts, same patient as in Figure 5-4. Photo courtesy of Kenneth G. Swan, MD.

abortion by gunshot was reported by Takki et al in 1969.[23] The woman's boyfriend deliberately shot her in the lower abdomen penetrating the uterus to abort the fetus. Fortunately the mother survived!

Exploration of gunshot wounds of the abdomen requires minute examination of all organs in the cavity. If one hole is present in the gut then a second hole must be looked for. Instances are often seen at the University Hospital in Newark where such second wounds are almost invisible as they are concealed along the mesenteric or omental borders. The colon-rectal area may need diagnostic studies postoperatively to locate the penetrating wounds, and a diverting colostomy is usually indicated when injury in the area is suspected due to blood in the rectum or the path of the bullet.

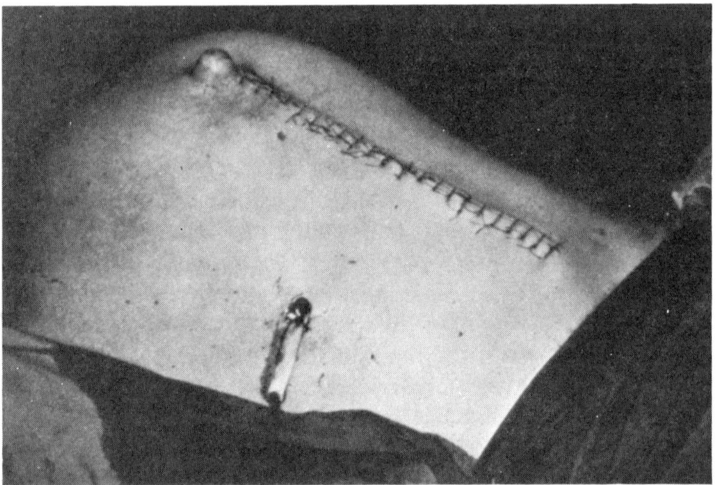

Figure 5-6 Closure of the abdomen after celiotomy and repair of perforation of stomach with bullet found in lesser sac. Reproduced with permission from Swan KG, Swan RC: *Gunshot Wounds.* Littleton, MA, PSG Publishing Co, Inc.

The use of prophylactic antibiotics is acceptable in gunshot wounds and the cephalosporins are the current drugs of choice. These are given intravenously either in the emergency department or in the operating room at the time of surgery and continued at least 48 hours postoperatively or longer if required by sepsis, adding secondary agents as indicated by culture and sensitivity studies.[24,25]

As with stab wounds, most gunshot wounds of the uterus can be repaired, but usually the uterus must be evacuated whether or not the patient is near term.

Cautious observation of the patient in whom ultrasonography, amniocentesis, and vital signs have demonstrated no fetal damage or distress after a low-velocity gunshot wound to the uterus may permit continuance of the pregnancy with the understanding that damage to the fetus may show up later on, usually resulting in spontaneous abortions, or perhaps requiring evacuation of the uterus once the fetus has died.

Gunshot wounds that involve body areas other than the abdomen may indirectly affect the outcome of the patient's pregnancy and are discussed in other chapters of the book. In general, penetrating wounds of the abdomen that penetrate the uterus may seriously jeopardize the life of the fetus.

REFERENCES

1. Chaim W, Mares AJ, Lieberman J, et al: Omental herniation: An unusual fetal complication of intrauterine transfusion. *Obstet Gynecol* 1976;47:621.
2. Haycock CE, Machiedo G: The use of peritoneal lavage as a diagnostic tool in emergencies. *J Am Coll Emerg Phys* 1974;397.
3. Freeark R: Penetrating wounds of the abdomen. *N Engl J Med* 1974; 291:185.
4. Cohn I: Surgical judgment in the management of penetrating wounds of the abdomen. *Ann Surg* 1974;179:639.
5. Robinson H: Application for laparoscopy in general surgery. *Surg Gynecol Obstet* 1976;143:829.
6. Gazzaniga A: Laparoscopy in the diagnosis of blunt and penetrating injuries to the abdomen. *Am J Surg* 1976;131:315.
7. Jordan G: Conservatism in the management of abdominal trauma. *Am J Surg* 1973;126:581.
8. Badia PD, Charleton A: Stab wound of a seven-month pregnant uterus. *NY State J Med* 1940;40:446.
9. Wright CH, Posner AC, Gilchrist J: Penetrating wounds of the gravid uterus. *Am J Obstet Gynecol* 1954;67:1085.
10. Quast DC, Jordan GL Jr: Traumatic wounds of the female reproductive organs. *J Trauma* 1964;4:839.
11. McNabney WK, Smith EI: Penetrating wounds of the gravid uterus. *J Trauma* 1972;12:1024.
12. Moss KL, Schmidt FE, Creech O: Analysis of 550 stab wounds of the abdomen. *Am Surg* 1962;28:483.
13. Dyer I, Barclay DL. Accidental trauma complicating pregnancy and delivery. *Am J Obstet Gynecol* 1962;83:907.
14. Lowe R: Should laparotomy be mandatory or selective in gunshot wounds of the abdomen. *J Trauma* 1977;17:903–907.
15. Browns K, Bhat R, Jonasson OL, et al: Thoracoabdominal gunshot wound with survival of a 36-week fetus. *JAMA* 1977;237:2409.

16. Gysler R, Haller R, Morger R: Intrauterine gunshot wound. *J Pediatr Surg* 1976;11:589.
17. Buchsbaum HJ: Diagnosis and management of abdominal gunshot wounds during pregnancy. *J Trauma* 1975;15:425.
18. Swan KG, Swan RC: *Gunshot Wounds*. Littleton, MA, PSG Publishing Co, Inc, 1980.
19. Wilson F, Swartz DP: Gunshot and war projectile wounds of the gravid uterus. Case report and review of literature. *J Natl Med Assoc* 1972;64:8.
20. Wray RC, Burnett WF: Gunshot wound of the intestine, pregnant uterus, and placenta with maternal and fetal survival. *Am Surg* 1971;37:308.
21. Buchsbaum HJ, Caruso PA: Gunshot wound of the pregnant uterus. *Obstet Gynecol* 1969;33:673.
22. Farzanfar M, Shell JH: Gunshot wound of the gravid uterus. *Am J Obstet Gynecol* 1966;95:877.
23. Takki S, Pollanen L, Ertama P, et al: Criminal abortion by gunshot. *Ann Chir Gynaecol Fenn* 1969;58:122.
24. Lord J: Prophylatic antibiotic wound irrigations in gastric, biliary and colonic surgery. *Am J Surg* 1983;145:209.
25. Neu H: Clinical uses of cephalosporins. *Lancet* 1982;2:252.

CHAPTER 6

BURNS AND OTHER TRAUMA IN PREGNANCY

CHRISTINE E. HAYCOCK

In the preceding chapters blunt and penetrating trauma have been discussed in detail, but there are other forms of trauma that require coverage. These include burns, asphyxiation, drowning, iatrogenic injuries, and self-induced damage associated with smoking, alcohol, and drugs. Burns will be addressed in some detail, and the other types of trauma will be briefly discussed.

BURNS

Despite the fact that over two million persons are burned per year, the number of pregnant women burned significantly enough to be admitted to hospitals is quite low. It has been calculated that about 5.7% of all women ages 15 to 39 years inclusive are pregnant at any one time according to British statistics published by their office of population census in 1980.

Statistics by Taylor et al in 1976,[1] Zhang et al in 1981,[2] and Matthews in 1982,[3] suggest that, although not frequent, burn injuries are not rare. Taking all their statistics into account, this would average out to about 0.06% of all pregnant women at any one time are burned severely enough to warrant hospital admission. There are undoubtedly many more pregnant women who suffer minor burns due to kitchen accidents, etc, while pregnant.

As with any other burn patient, the prognosis of the pregnant woman depends upon the extent of the burn. An early report by Ryan et al in 1972,[4] had suggested that pregnancy might have increased the patient's survival from burns, but this has been shown to be fallacious.

On the other hand, the chances of survival of the fetus are diminished. Spontaneous abortion in the first trimester of pregnancy may go unnoticed or be put aside as trivial, but fetal death in the second trimester is usually 99% in severe burns, and survival in the third trimester is rare unless immediate delivery occurs (or caesarean section is carried out) within five days of injury.[3]

Before further discussion of these topics, a review of burn care should be presented for the benefit of those who do not deal with such care on a frequent basis.

Initial care requires an immediate estimation of the extent and depth of the burn. Clothing must be completely removed. (Do not pull adherent clothing off burned skin as this may increase damage. Place the patient or part in a warm saline soak or tub and let the stuck cloth come loose spontaneously.)

Pain may be safely treated with intravenous narcotics as required and poses no problem immediately to the fetus, although it should be noted at time of delivery if this event occurs in the early burn period.

The rule of nines (Table 6-1) will quickly determine the percentage of burn, and the depth of burn can be fairly well determined by visual and tactile determination (Table 6-2). Patients with burns of over 15% second degree, or 5% third

Table 6-1
Rule of Nines for Burns in Adults

Head	9%	
Each Arm	9%	(Total 18%)
Each Leg	18%	(Total 36%)
Anterior Trunk	18%	
Posterior Trunk	18%	
Genitals and Perineum	1%	

Table 6-2
Types of Burns

First Degree:
Skin pink or red (sunburn), soft, sensitive to touch, hair intact.

Second Degree:
Skin red with blisters, partial thickness involved, hair may be singed but present. Very painful to the touch. Skin is soft, pliable, but elevated.

Third Degree:
Two Depths

A. Almost full thickness of skin involved. Hair gone, white with thrombosed vessels often seen, leathery feel, insensitive to touch but pressure felt. Little pain.

B. Full thickness skin down to bone possible. Brown, often charred. No sensation, painless. Muscle, nerves, vessels and tendons may be gone.

degree, or those with burns which involve the eyes, ears, face, hands, or perineum usually require at least initial hospitalization. Major burns are defined as those over 25% second degree, over 10% third degree, or complicated by other injuries or disease. (Burns of 15% to 25% second degree are considered moderate burns.) Pregnancy per se does not change these classifications.

Once the percent and severity of the burn has been quickly determined definitive treatment must begin, but because of the fetus's susceptibility to anoxia, any evidence of smoke inhalation should be treated by immediate use of nasal oxygen for the safety of both mother and fetus.

A history of unconsciousness at any time during the fire or exposure to smoke in a closed room may be considered presumptive evidence of smoke inhalation. Clinical examination of the face and oropharynx may reveal visual evidence of soot, singed nasal hairs, or facial burns. Auscultation of the chest may reveal rales, rhonchi, or wheezes, the patient may be coughing up soot-stained sputum and may show hoarseness when she speaks. Radiologic evidence may lag behind these findings several hours.[5]

Immediate blood gases should be obtained along with the normal blood studies obtained in all burn patients (complete blood cell count, electrolytes, etc). Intravenous fluids are given according to the usual formulas such as the Parkland formula, in which no colloid is given in the first 24 hours and crystalloids such as Ringer's lactate or sodium chloride solutions at the rate of 4 mL/kg/% body burn in the first 24 hours and then adjusted as needed by serum chemical and electrolyte determinations.

Urinary output in the pregnant burn patient should be monitored closely during the acute burn period and maintained at least 30–50 mL per hour (or at 100 mL per hour if using the Parkland formula). The increased maternal volume need not be considered in this respect.

Fluid loss is greatest in the first 12 hours, but the hypovolemic shock period generally persists over a 36-hour period so that constant replacement is required. British physicians tend to use colloid solutions such as human freeze-dried plasma more often than do physicians in the United States.

Direct treatment of the burned areas are also routine in the pregnant burn patient. Surgery may be carried out if required for early excision of third-degree burns or removal of eschars as required. "Early" usually means about the fourth post burn day. "Late" surgery usually refers to grafting done about three weeks post burn.

The burn area is generally treated with topical application of antibacterial creams such as silver sulfadiazine (Silvadene) after debridement and cleansing baths as indicated daily. Antibiotics are used systemically only to prevent secondary infection such as pneumonia, especially when lung damage from smoke inhalation may have occurred.

Nutritional requirements are important as meeting the increased metabolic needs after trauma will also allow an increased metabolic responsiveness. With increased availability of amino acids, greater protein synthesis and less protein degradation are likely. This will improve the body defenses of the burn patient to infection which is the major cause of mortality to these patients. Their immune protection tends to be compromised, and bacterial invasion with septicemia then results.[6]

Survival of patients with greater than 50% body burns is poor in any group of burn patients, but it is dismal in pregnant patients in the second or third trimesters. The statistics are about the same for those in the first trimester as in the nonpregnant patient, but fetal survival is lower.

Matthews in his study of 50 patients,[3] and Zhang et al in their study of 24 patients,[2] showed not only that maternal survival is poor, but also that the fetus may well be lethal to the mother with a burn greater than 50% if not delivered within a few hours of the burn injury. The babies survived in two cases at 5 and 8 days, but the mothers died.

Because the maternal plasma volume increases by up to 50% with peripheral vasodilatation as pregnancy progresses, the pregnant patient is less able to adapt to the stress on her cardiovascular system posed by sepsis in the third trimester as she is already close to the limits of cardiovascular tolerance. Only the rapid delivery of the fetus which results in a return to normal of plasma volume within 6 to 8 weeks and especially in the first few days post delivery, will help. The hypercoagulable state seen during pregnancy also swiftly returns to normal.[3]

Thus, rapid delivery in the second and third trimesters may result in maternal survival even though the fetus is lost, and this procedure is advocated by either induced labor or caesarean section for patients with greater than 50% burns.

A few cases of major burns in early pregnancy have occurred with survival of mother and fetus.[4,7] When possible, spasmolytic agents can be tried to suppress labor. A suggestion that the antiprostaglandins might be of some value in preventing abortion by prostaglandin PGE_2 stimulation has been made following studies by Karim et al in 1971,[8] and Stage in 1973.[9]

Fetal survival must take a secondary role to maternal survival, although every attempt should be made by rapid delivery by induction or caesarean section to save a viable infant while also aiding the severely burned mother. The fetus produces nonspecific antibodies that block the activity of the maternal lymphocytes, resulting in the patient being more susceptible antigenically to infection and its severe consequences in late pregnancy. Estrogen levels are thought to play a role in morbidity also.[10]

Other problems also face the burned pregnant patient after delivery and recovery from the burn. Severe chest area burns may result in loss of the nipples and therefore the inability of the mother to nurse her infant.[11,12] This can also result in tender swollen breast tissues until the glandular activity is dried up due to lack of stimulation, and any medications used to reduce milk production.

The woman with a severely burned abdominal wall also faces problems because of the loss of the normal ability of the abdominal skin to stretch. This causes problems that worsen as the patient approaches term.[11-15] The patient experiences tautness and a burning sensation of the skin, which can result in loss of sleep and interfere with normal daily activities. This can result in a need to hospitalize the patient where bed rest, sedation, and inactivity ameliorate the symptoms.

Most reported patients have carried to term, but in a few reported instances,[11,13,14] labor was induced early because of severe pain. There does not appear to be an increased incidence of abortion associated with this problem.

LIGHTNING

There have been about a dozen cases of lightning striking pregnant women reported in the literature.[16-19] This rare event has resulted in the loss of the fetus, even though the mother survived in about 50% of the cases.

Labor is believed to be induced if there is passage of high-voltage current through the uterus. If pregnancy is near term this is more apt to occur. Rupture of the uterus due to the severity of the contractions has been reported. Both the amniotic fluid and uterus are said to be good conductors of electric current. If this current strikes the fetus, cardiac arrest results.[20]

The pregnant patient may be rendered unconscious and require cardiopulmonary resuscitation. This effort should not be abandoned too early, as fixed and dilated pupils do not in this instance always indicate death.[20]

No resuscitation of the fetus in utero has so far been attempted, but one author[17] speculated that this may be worthy of investigation. One case has been reported in the literature,[21] of a long-term follow-up of a survivor of an intrauterine lightning strike. In this instance the fetus was delivered without incident and was a healthy male.

CARBON MONOXIDE INHALATION

Although air polution from industry and automobiles produces most carbon monoxide, it is the insidiously inhaled variety from cigarette smoking that is of greatest concern to the pregnant woman.

Numerous reports now in the literature have reported its dangerous effects. Copel et al[22] report decreased fetal birth weight directly related to the number of cigarettes smoked. Other reported effects are increased fetal loss, abruptio placenta, placenta previa, and premature rupture of membranes. Demonstrated late effects such as decreased mental abilities and height as well as hyperkinetic children are reported in a large British study and others.[23]

The transplacental passage of carbon monoxide to the fetus in utero has been demonstrated by many studies, past and present. The results of this crossing unfortunately may not become evident for months or years.[24]

An interesting report was of an accidental death of the fetus by carbon monoxide poisoning due to a faulty gas valve on a kitchen stove. The patient, who was in her third trimester of pregnancy, was found in the morning by relatives with headache, fatigue, lethargy, stomach cramps, and a rapid heart rate. She was treated by 100% oxygen by a nonrebreathing mask which dropped her COHg from 23.7% to 1.7%, but sonography revealed the absence of fetal heart tones. Induced labor with prostaglandin E delivered a macerated, stillborn infant. Tissue analysis of liver and spleen revealed a 31.5% COHg.[25]

The only treatment is prevention. Get pregnant women to stop smoking! The socioeconomic consequences must be consistently published.

ENVIRONMENTAL AND OCCUPATIONAL HAZARDS

As more and more pregnant women enter the labor market, particularly in more nontraditional jobs such as mining and industrial labor, they become exposed to toxic industrial hazards during pregnancy. One environmental example was the teratogenic effects seen in Japan of methyl mercury contaminated fish consumed by women workers.

In industry, lead-related jobs may pose a hazard.[26] Lead is widely used as an industrial chemical and has been reported to cause increased rates of spontaneous abortion, perinatal mortality, mental retardation and neonatal convulsions.

Polychlorinated biphenyls have been used for years in electric transformers, capacitors, hydraulic fluids, lubricants, and carbonless copy paper. Infants have developed hyperpigmentation, slowed behavioral development, and increased neonatal mortality.[26]

Heat stress is another occupational concern in nontraditional jobs in hot areas. This may result in compounding the cardiovascular stress normally present in pregnancy. Increased stillbirths with resorption or decreased birth weight may result.[27]

CAFFEINE AND OTHER DRUGS

Although no human malformation has been directly attributed to the consumption of caffeine, a daily intake of more than

600 mg has been associated with human fetal death and birth defects.[28] This generally results from the consumption of over 8 cups of coffee per day, and the caffeine intake may be enhanced by ingestion of over-the-counter drugs and caffeinated soft drinks. Animal studies have been more positive in revealing direct caffeine effects than human studies, but certainly reduction of high caffeine intake in pregnant women in advisable.

Other toxicity reports indicate problems with drugs such as Bendectin (dicyclomine hydrochloride, doxylamine succinate, and pyridoxine), used for morning sickness,[29] diazepam (Valium), phenytoin (Dilantin) and other antiepileptic drugs, and excessive doses of progesterone compounds.[30,31]

ALCOHOL

Alcohol definitely contributes to trauma inasmuch as statistics indicate that intoxication is involved in over 50% of all fatal motor vehicle accidents, however, heavy alcohol ingestion by the pregnant patient causes direct effects on the developing fetus.

A study by Halliday et al[32] in Ireland revealed that about one third of the offspring of chronic alcoholic mothers had obvious abnormalities termed the fetal alcohol syndrome (Jones and Smith[33]). Some of the results are poor growth, transient neurological disturbances, and abnormal facies. Breech presentation and birth asphyxia with hypoglycemia and polycytemia are also more common.

Many studies have been done on this problem recently and the American Medical Association published an extensive Council on Scientific Affairs report of the subject.[34] Other studies by Little and Streissguth[35] and Sokol[36] verified the findings, and the counseling of pregnant women on the adverse effects of alcohol and other agents is advised.[37]

IATROGENIC INJURIES

With the increase of the use of intrapartum fetal monitoring it is anticipated that iatrogenic injuries may occur due to the use of the aspirating needles or electrodes to either mother or fetus. One such case has been reported and more probably have occurred that have not been reported. The reported case by Akhter[38] was a second-degree scalp burn caused by a spinal electrode used during intrapartum fetal monitoring.

SUMMARY

A large amount of material has been briefly reviewed in this chapter, and the reader is advised to research the applicable reference materials if further detail is desired. Other aspects of trauma in pregnancy are covered in more detail in other chapters of the book.

REFERENCES

1. Taylor JW, Plunkett GD, McManus W, et al: Thermal injury during pregnancy. *Obstet Gynecol* 1976;47:434.
2. Zhang YB, Wang XW, Zhang YJ, et al: Burns during pregnancy. Analysis of 24 cases. *Chinese Med J* 1981;94:123.
3. Matthews RN: Obstetric implications of burns in pregnancy. *Br J Obstet Gynaecol* 1982;89:603.
4. Ryan RF, Longenecker CG, Vincent RW: Effects of pregnancy on healing of burns. *Surg Forum Am Coll Surg* 1962;13:483.
5. Greenberg MI: Axioms on smoke inhalation. *Hosp Med* March 1983;23.
6. Alexander JW: Host defense mechanisms after injury, *Proceedings from the Metabolic and Nutrition Support for Trauma and Burn Patients Symposium.* 17 July 1982, p 3.
7. Stillwell JH: A major burn in early pregnancy with maternal survival and pregnancy progressing to term. *Br J Plast Surg* 1982; 35:33.
8. Karim SMM, Hillier K, Somers K, et al: The effects of prostaglandins E_2 and F_2 alpha administered by different routes on uterine activity and the cardiovascular system in pregnant and non-pregnant women. *J Obstet Gynaecol Br Commonw* 1971;78:172.
9. Stage AH: Severe burns in the pregnant patient. *Obstet Gynecol* 1973;42:259.
10. Harkness RA: Oestrogens and host resistance. *J Roy Soc Med* 1980; 73:161.

11. Daw E, Mohandas I: Pregnancy in patients after severe abdominal burns. *Br J Obstet Gynaecol* 1983;90:69.
12. Trott JA, Hobby JAE: Burns of the female breast; a long term study. *Burns* 1978;4:267.
13. Haeseker B, Green MF: A complication in pregnancy due to severe burns in childhood. *Br Plast Surg* 1981;34:102.
14. Rai YS, Jackson DM: Child-bearing in relation to the scarred abdominal wall from burns. *Burns* 1975;1:167,
15. Matthews RN: Old burns and pregnancy. *Br J Obstet Gynaecol* 1982;89:610.
16. Weinstein L: Lightning: A rare cause of intrauterine death with maternal survival. *Southern Med J* 1979;72:632.
17. Guha-Ray DK: Fetal death at term due to lightning. *Am J Obstet Gynecol* 79; 134:103.
18. Rees WD: Pregnant woman struck by lightning. *Br Med J* 1965; 1:103.
19. Chan YF, Sivasamboo R: Lightning accident in pregnancy. *J Obstet Gynaecol Br Common* 1972;79:761.
20. Apfelberg DB, Masters FW, Robinson DW: Pathophysiology and treatment of lightning injuries. *J Trauma* 1974;l4:453.
21. Flannery DB, Wiles H: Follow-up of a survivor of intrauterine lightning exposure. *Am J Obstet Gynecol* 1982;142:238.
22. Copel JA, Bowen F, Bolognese RJ: Carbon monoxide intoxication in early pregnancy. *Obstet Gynecol* 1982;59:26S.
23. Longo LD: The biological effects of carbon monoxide on the pregnant woman, fetus, and newborn infant. *Am J Obstet Gynecol* 1977;129:69.
24. Longo LD: Carbon monoxide in the pregnant mother and fetus and its exchange across the placenta. *Ann NY Acad Sci* 1970,174:313.
25. Cramer CR: Fetal death due to accidental maternal carbon monoxide poisoning. *J Toxicol Clin Toxicol* 1982,19:297.
26. Brix KA: Environmental and occupational hazards to the fetus. *J Repro Med* 1982;17:577.
27. Edwards MJ: Is hyperthermia a human teratogen? *Am Heart J* 1979; 98:277.
28. Brooten D, Jordan CH: Caffeine and pregnancy. A research review and recommendations for clinical practice. *JOGN Nursing* l983; 12:190.
29. Evans AN, Brooke OG, West RJ: The ingestion by pregnant women of substances toxic to the foetus. *Practitioner* 1980;224:315.
30. Bartoshesky LE, Bhan I, Nagpaul K, et al: Severe cardiac and ophthalmologic malformations in an infant exposed to diphenylhydantoin in utero. *Pediatrics* 1982;69:202.

31. Kullander S, Kahlen B, Sandahl B: Exposure to drugs and other possibly harmful factors during the first trimester of pregnancy. Comparison of two prospective studies performed in Sweden 10 years apart. *Acta Obstet Gynecol Scand* 1976;55:395.
32. Halliday HL, Reid MM, McClure G: Results of heavy drinking in pregnancy. *Br J Obstet Gynaecol* 1982;89:892.
33. Jones KL, Smith DW: Recognition of the fetal alcohol syndrome in early infancy. *Lancet* 1973;2:999.
34. Council Report: Fetal effects of maternal alcohol use. *JAMA* 1983;249:2517.
35. Little RE, Streissguth AP: Effects of alcohol on the fetus: Impact and prevention. *Can Med Assoc J* 1981,125:159.
36. Sokol RJ: Alcohol and abnormal outcomes of pregnancy. *Can Med Assoc J* 1981;125:143.
37. Shepard TH: Counseling pregnant women exposed to potentially harmful agents during pregnancy. *Clin Obstet Gynecol* 1983; 26:478.
38. Akhter MS: An unusual complication of intrapartum fetal monitoring. *Am J Obstet Gynecol* 1976;124:657.

CHAPTER 7

PREGNANCY AND RADIOGRAPHIC EXAMINATION

GAIL ELIOT
DANDAMUDI V. RAO

In managing the traumatized female patient of child-bearing age, consideration of pregnancy should always be present. After identifying the pregnant patient or with a patient suspected of being pregnant, the decision to proceed with radiographic studies will be made weighing the potential hazard of the procedure against the hazard of not performing the procedure. The known effects of radiation on the developing fetus will be discussed, as well as the estimated dose for various x-ray studies. Decisions and recommendations can then be based upon knowledge of facts.

CLINICAL AND BIOLOGIC CONSIDERATIONS

Identifying the pregnant patient is not easy. Most unsuspected pregnancies are within the first few weeks of conception. Since the most sensitive time for radiation damage is also at this time, the problem of identifying the gravid patient takes on special importance. Six percent (6%) of the female population of child-bearing age is pregnant. Two percent (2%) are in their first trimester. About half of these pregnancies, 1% of women in the child-bearing population, are unknown to the gravida. Elective radiographic studies can be scheduled up to 10 days after the last normal menstrual cycle to avoid unsuspected pregnancy. But emergency examinations associated with trauma may not be avoided, but can be modified.

It has been recommended that a beta subunit radioimmunoassay test for pregnancy be performed routinely to identify early pregnancy when x-ray of the pelvis is contemplated. This test will be positive as early as one week after conception or one week after the missed period.[1] The problem associated with this is a practical one. Most hospitals do not have the test available on an emergency basis 24 hours a day. Ultrasound examination would also reveal changes associated with pregnancy 3–4 weeks after ovulation. It is prudent to assume that a patient of child bearing age may be pregnant, as there is a potential for damage to the fetus, starting in the last few days before the expected menstrual cycle. If a beta-subunit is available, it should be utilized. If it is not available, modifications of studies and avoidance of fluoroscopy should be practiced.

The earliest reports of fetal damage due to intrauterine radiation exposure were made by Murphy[2] and Goldstein,[3] who studied the records of 106 women who received therapeutic doses of radiation during pregnancy. Seventy-five term births resulted in 38 abnormal children. Twenty-eight of the abnormal children had defects clearly attributable to the radiation. These included 16 microcephalics, two with normal head size but mentally retarded, and one hydrocephalic. Additional anomalies of the spine, skeletal system and blindness were observed.[4]

After the atomic bomb attacks on Hiroshima and Nagasaki, studies were made of the women who were pregnant and exposed at the time of the attack. Plummer reported a study of 205 4.5-year-old children who had been exposed during the first half of intrauterine life in Hiroshima.[5] Eleven were exposed within 1200 meters of the bomb hypocenter. Seven had microcephaly with mental retardation. None of the children outside this zone had microcephaly. Other anomalies had no greater incidence than expected in the general population. Yamazaki and Wright reported on the experience in Nagasaki.[6] This study differed in that evaluation of the entire time of the pregnancy was included and the area of study was limited at 2000 meters from the bomb hypocenter. There were 30 mothers who experienced symptoms of major radiation exposure (epilation, oropharyngeal lesions, purpura, or petechiae) and who were within the 2000 meters.

There were seven fetal deaths and six neonatal and infant deaths. Of the surviving children, four were mentally retarded. One mother was exposed in the first trimester, two were in the second trimester and one was exposed in the third trimester. The height head circumference of the surviving children were significantly smaller than those of controls.

A review of all reports of human radiation exposure in utero was done by Dekaban in 1968.[7] Out of over 200 cases reported in the literature, only 26 had sufficient information to be able to calculate dose and gestational age. In this group of 26, doses ranged from 250 rads to many thousand. At 3 weeks to 12 weeks of gestational age multiple organ defects were produced in addition to microcephaly. Six fetuses exposed at 10 to 20 weeks of gestational age had microcephaly and stunted growth. Three fetuses exposed after 19 weeks of gestational age had no abnormality. The most frequent abnormalities were 1) small size at birth and stunted growth, 2) microcephaly, 3) mental retardation, 4) microphthalmus, 5) pigmentary degeneration of the retina, 6) genital and skeletal malformations and 7) cataracts. The evidence thus obtained is in agreement with experimental studies conducted on mice (see below).

There are three distinct phases of radiation damage related to gestational age. The three stages are preimplantation, organogenesis, and fetal stage. During preimplantation and early implantation there is a high incidence of embryo deaths. As little as 5 rads to 15 rads in mice can cause death,[8] but those cells and embryos that survive are totipotential and continue to develop normally. This stage in man is less than 3 weeks of gestational age. The primitive streak stage is around 16 gestational days,[7] and this is beyond the totipotential stage for surviving cells.

Organogenesis is the second phase. There are fewer fetal deaths in this stage, and more anomalies are produced. The neural tube begins to form at about 22 or 23 gestational days. As the structures of the brain progress from a single cerebral vesicle at 4 weeks to an expanded and differentiated cerebral cortex at 20 weeks, the anomalies produced will reflect the stage of development at which time the radiation was delivered. So, at 3 to 7 weeks of gestation, exencephaly, dysraphism, single cerebral ventricle, hydrocephaly and hypoplastic and small brain may occur. At approximately 8 to 16 weeks, cellular deficit, heterotopias, deformities of various structures, or generally small brain, sometimes associated with secondary dilitation of the ventricles, occurs. At 17 to 24 weeks mild cortical abnormalities and slightly reduced size of the brain are recorded. Additionally, other organ systems are affected during organogenesis. Skeletal abnormalities, genital abnormalities, retinal pigmentation, and cataracts are associated with radiation in the 3rd to 11th gestational weeks.[7]

After the completion of organogenesis, in the fetal stage, deficits are more likely to be functional and less obvious to the observer. There is a somewhat arbitrary cutoff for the end of organogenesis and the beginning of the fetal stage at 16 weeks. But this should not be mistaken to mean that after 16 weeks it is safe. The differentiating cells are still sensitive, and potential central nervous system damage continues throughout pregnancy and into postnatal life. Neuroblasts are probably found in the human embryo from about 16 days postconception until about two weeks after birth. Neuroblasts are so radiosensitive that they can be destroyed by 25 rads.[7] This is confirmed by a spastic child born of an atomic bomb victim who was in her last trimester.[2]

In summary, radiation damage during the preimplantation stage causes embryo death or no damage (about the time of, or a few days before, the first missed period). Damage during organogenesis of skeletal and genital systems results in anomalies from 3 to 16 weeks. Microcephaly and central nervous system functional abnormalities continue to 20 weeks and beyond.

Most of the human data are based upon high therapeutic doses of radiation or large doses received in an atomic bomb blast. How can this be applied to diagnostic doses? As mentioned above, Rugh reported kill of the fertilized rodent egg and gross anomalies of the rodent central nervous system at 5 to 15 rads.[8] The lowest human radiation dose resulting in microcephaly was 10 to 19 rads in air to a mother in Hiroshima,[9] but the exposure consisted of 20% neutrons and 80% gamma rays. Neutrons have a high linear energy transfer which makes them biologically more damaging. Gamma rays and x-rays are identical at the same energy. Gamma rays result from natural decay, whereas x-rays (Roentgen rays) are generated from an x-ray tube. Other experimental data on low dose irradiation of mice have been reported by various investigators.[10] Russell, in studying effects on the skeletal systems, found that the lowest dose to yield radiation effects was 25 rads.[11] This affected 0% to 20% of survivors during organogenesis. The overall effect on skeletal development at 10 rads should be indistinguishable from randomly occurring anomalies. Brent reports on increased incidence of malformation rate in mice and rats at 20 rads given at the time of the primitive streak.[9] Noting that the excess risk of adverse effects arising from doses below 10 rad to the human embryo-fetus are considered by many to represent an acceptable risk when compared to the potential medical benefit of the examination to the patient.[9]

What type of studies are likely to be necessary in the traumatized patient? For studies that do not include the uterus in the direct beam the dose delivered to the fetus is negligible if appropriate columnation of the beam and shielding are used. Trauma studies that will include the uterus in the direct beam include examination of the pelvis, hips, lumbar spine, sacrum, coccyx, abdomen, intravenous pyelogram, cystogram, myelogram, and pelvic angiography. Computerized tomography (CT) recently been added to evaluate for visceral injuries, splenic injury, acetabular fractures, and spine injury. Modification of these examinations can be done so that only one or two exposures are necessary for pelvis, hips, spine, sacrum, abdomen, intravenous pyelogram, and cystogram. X-ray of the coccyx probably is not justified, as a fracture will not alter patient management. This will provide a dose of under 2 rads for these studies. A word about hip examinations. The uterus can be carefully shielded from the direct beam without shielding the hip, but this is difficult if not done meticulously. The result will be an unsatisfactory study if the hip is also shielded, and repeat exposure will be required. Pelvic angiography may be necessary to define and treat hemorrhage from pelvic fractures. Fluoroscopy should be as limited as possible. This is the occasion for an experienced angiographer. Use of video playback equipment may also allow the radiologist more viewing time without repeated exposures and test injections. A record should be made of the fluoroscopy time and number of films so that an accurate dose can be calculated (by the hospital's medical physicist later). A dosimeter could also be placed directly on the patient's skin to measure skin dose. The dose is about 3 rads per slice. Sequential slices made by moving the patient on the CT table programmed increments, avoiding overlap, and even allowing a small gap between slices, will result in a 3-rad dose to any volume to tissue directly irradiated. If, however, there are contiguous slices, the dose will be about twice as much or 6 rads to any volume due to scatter from adjacent slices. In spine trauma, a myelogram can be avoided by use of computerized tomography alone or CT with a small intrathecal dose of metrizimide to provide contrast. This has a potentially lower dose than a myelogram, which requires fluoroscopy as well as films.

Emergency x-ray studies involving the pelvis therefore can be performed with doses below 5 rads if the study is modified. CT should be performed with thin slices allowing for gaps between slices. The possible exception is angiography for pelvic hemorrhage. This study will most likely result in a dose greater than 5 rads. Since this is a life-threatening situation, the study will have to be performed. Accurate records of dose should be made at the time of study to permit informed decision making regarding the risk to the fetus.

RADIATION PHYSICS CONSIDERATIONS

The unit of radiation dose is the rad, which is defined as the energy absorption of 100 ergs per g of any material. Recently the International Commission on Radiation Units has recommended the use of the gray (Gy), which is defined as 1 J of energy absorption in 1 kg of matter, as the new unit for radiation dose. For those who are used to the old unit of radiation dose, the conversion factor is 1 Gy = 100 rads. Since 1 erg is equal to 6.24×10^5 MeV, the absorbed dose is 1 rad when 1 g of matter receives 6.24×10^7 MeV of energy (1 eV is by definition equal to the energy required by an electron falling through a potential difference of 1 V). One Gy is therefore equal to an energy absorption of 6.24×10^9 MeV in 1 g of matter.

It is well known that 1 Gy of radiation dose from protons, neutrons, or alpha particles is more damaging than the same dose from gamma rays, x-rays, or electrons. Because of this difference in quality of different radiations, another unit of dose equivalent is defined, and it is known as rem in the old system. In the SI system, it is called the Sievert (Sv), which is the dose equivalent for an absorbed dose of 1 Gy if the equality factor is 1. Thus, 1 Sv = 100 rems. If the quality factor is more than one, as the case of protons, neutrons, and alpha particles, the dose equivalent to Sieverts is equal to quality factor times the absorbed dose in Grays.

For the purpose of describing radiation levels in a radiation area, another unit for exposure is needed and it is known as roentgen (R). In the old system of units, this is defined as the ionization producing an amount of charge equal to 2.58×10^{-4} C/kg of air, about 2×10^9 ion pairs per cubic centimeter of dry air at standard temperature and pressure. The SI unit for exposure is the C/kg, which is approximately equal to 3875 R.

MAXIMUM PERMISSIBLE DOSES

It is impossible not to receive any radiation exposure. We all receive a radiation dose of 0.1 rem per year, or an exposure level of about 100 mR per year. This is the background level resulting primarily from natural radiation sources and cosmic radiation. It will vary from place to place depending on the latitude and altitude.

For the purposes of discussion, the maximum permissible doses (MPD) to individuals can be divided into four categories. (These recommendations are made by the National Council on Radiation Protection [NCRP Report No.39] and are generally accepted by the various regulatory agencies. In what follows, we will discuss the method to estimate the dose to the fetus from medical x-ray exposures to pregnant women.)

Occupational Workers

Occupational workers are those required to work with radiation-producing machines as part of their jobs. The recommended MPD for whole body, gonads, lens of the eyes and bone marrow is 5 rem in any one year, and the MPD for accumulated occupational dose to the whole body should not exceed $5(N - 18)$ where N is the person's age in years. For a 30-year-old person, the MPD is $5(30 - 18) = 5 \times 12 = 60$ rem. The allowed MPD for skin, hands and forearms is 15, 75, and 30 rems per year, respectively. For all other organs it is 15 rems per year.

Nonoccupational Workers

The recommended limit for whole body dose for persons in this category is 0.5 rem per year.

Medical Exposures

The above limits for occupational and nonoccupational workers does not include any required medical exposures. The only limitation for medical exposures is that the benefit to the patient must outweigh the risk associated with the exposure.

Pregnant Women and Fetus

The MPD to the fetus of an expectant mother is 0.5 rem. The lower limit to the fetus is understandable considering the fact that it is most sensitive to radiation.

DOSE TO THE FETUS FROM X-RAY PROCEDURES

Since the mammalian organism is most sensitive to radiation during the intrauterine stages of development, the National Council on Radiation Protection recommends that the physician exercise special care in patient selection in the case of women of child-bearing age. In the best judgment of the physician, if it is necessary to perform the radiographic or nuclear medicine examination for the medical well-being of the patient without delay, the physician should know the dose that the fetus and the possibly pregnant woman will receive and its effects.

The dose to the uterus from x-ray procedures depends on several factors: 1) x-ray tube potential (kVp), 2) current (mA), 3) exposure time (s), 4) filtration, 5) size of the patient, 6) type of procedure or projections, 7) source-to-film distance, and 8) type of x-ray generator. It is therefore obvious one cannot estimate the dose to the fetus from just the type of examination without knowing the above-mentioned parameters.

Table 7-1 provides an estimated dose to the embryo for selected x-ray projections. In calculating the dose to an average-sized woman, we have assumed that the x-ray machine used has a three-phase generator and the filtration is 2.5 mm of Al and that the source to film distance is 100 m. The dose to the fetus is approximate and varies depending on the parameters used on conducting the x-ray examination. It is suggested that the institution's medical physicist be consulted for more accurate dose estimates for a given exposure setup, particularly when the knowledge of the fetus dose is important for the overall assessment of the patient care.

Table 7-1
Embryo Doses for Selected X-ray Projections

Projection	View	kVp	mA	Image Receptor Size (in inches)	Dose (M rad per Radiograph)
Pelvic, lumbo-	AP	80	60	17 × 14	357
pelvic	Lat	80	60	14 × 17	50
Lumbar spine	AP	120	80	14 × 17	1260
	Lat	120	80	14 × 17	204
Full spine	AP	80	90	14 × 36	729
Hip (both)	AP	80	60	17 × 14	450
Femur	AP	80	60	7 × 17	5
Abdominal*	AP	80	90	14 × 17	503
	PA	80	90	14 × 17	250
	Lat	80	90	14 × 17	75
Renalomogram	AP	70	50	10 × 12	192
Cystography					
Upper GI	AP	120	75	14 × 17	162
Cholecystography	PA	80	90	10 × 12	5.5
Chest	AP	140	10	14 × 17	2.6
Barium swallow	AP	90	25	14 × 17	0.6
Ribs	AP	70	40	14 × 17	0.3
Thoracic spine	AP	80	90	14 × 17	1.9
Skull, Cervical spine, scapula, shoulder, humerus					0.01
CT Abdomen 2800 mA 110 kVp (if the fetus is included in the slice.)					

*Includes barium enema, lumbosacral spine, IVP, pyelogram, KUB, renal arteriogram.
kVp = kilovolt (peak); mA = milliamperes per second.

REFERENCES

1. Syed IB, Samols E: Medical x-ray exposure of the human embryo and fetus. *Health Phys* 1982;42:61.
2. Murphy DP: The outcome of 625 pregnancies in women subjected

to pelvic radium or roentgen irradiation. *Am J Obstet Gynecol* 1929;18:179.

3. Goldstein L: Radiogenic microcephaly-survey of nineteen recorded cases, with special reference to opththalmic defects. *Arch Neurol Psych* 1930;24:102.
4. Hall EJ: *Radiobiology for the Radiologist*. New York, Harper & Row, 1973, p 213.
5. Plummer G: Anomalies occuring in children exposed in utero to the atomic bomb in Hiroshima. *Pediatrics* 1952;10:687-693.
6. Yamazaki J, Wright S, Wright P: Outcome of pregnancy in women exposed to the atomic bomb in Nagasaki. *Am J Dis Child* 1954; 87:448.
7. Dekaban A: Abnormalities in children exposed to x-radiation during various stages of gestation: Tentative timetable of radiation injury to the human fetus, part I. *J Nuclear Med* 1968;9:471.
8. Rugh R: Low levels of x-irradiation and early mammalian embryo. *Am J Roentgenol* 1962;87:559.
9. Rugh R: The impact of ionizing radiations on the embryo and fetus. *Am J Roentgenol* 1963;89:182.
10. Hall EJ: Page 232 and NCRP Report No. 54, p 5. (Original article by Russell LB: Effects of low doses of x-rays on embryonic development in the mouse. *Proc Soc Exp Biol Med* 1957;95:174.)
11. Russell LB: Effects of low doses of x-ray on embryonic development in the mouse. *Proc Soc Exp Biol Med* 1957;95:174.

CHAPTER 8

ANESTHETIC MANAGEMENT OF THE TRAUMATIZED PARTURIENT

MAKRAM ERIAN
WEN-HSIEN WU

In clinical management of a traumatized parturient one must consider the well-being of both mother and fetus. Thus, understanding the anatomic and physiologic alterations during pregnancy is essential.[1-3] To interpret properly the clinical signs and diagnostic studies commonly employed in the management of trauma, these alterations affecting nearly every organ system in early pregnancy, which are largely due to hormonal factors and later on to physiologic adaption to the growing gravid uterus and its mechanical effects, must be kept in mind as detailed in Chapter 1 and as reiterated below.

In the cardiovascular system both blood volume and the blood constituents begin to increase from the 12th week of gestation and reach the maximum by the 32nd week and remain at that level until term. After delivery they begin to decline. At term the plasma volume increases by 40% to 50% of the normal values. The fibrinogen level and platelets increase similarly during the course of gestation and thus predispose to thromboembolic states. The gradually increasing cardiac output with decreased peripheral vascular resistance reaches its peak of 50% above normal at 32 weeks.

In the respiratory system the anatomical changes, including vascular congestion of the upper airways, increased antero-posterior and transverse diameters of the thoracic cage, and diaphragmatic elevation, contribute to the changes in lung volumes. Beginning from the 20th week, the expiratory reserve volume and functional residual capacity are decreasing. However, with an concomitant increase in inspiratory capacity and inspiratory reserve volume the total lung capacity remains unchanged. At term the functional residual capacity is reduced by 20% of normal. The total airway resistance is reduced due to progesterone-induced relaxation of the bronchial smooth muscles. The minute ventilation begins to increase as early as the 10th to 12th week, reaching 50% above the normal. Maternal hyperventilation during pregnancy leads to an increase of PaO_2 to a mean value of 106 to 110 torr (formerly abbreviated mmHg), with a reduction of $PaCO_2$ to a mean of 32 torr. To compensate for the hypocapnia the kidneys excrete base to normalize the pH. However, this results in a decrease of plasma buffer base.

The gastrointestinal tract shows delayed gastric emptying. This is a result of progesterone-induced relaxation of gastric smooth muscles and mechanical displacement of the pylorus by the growing gravid uterus.[1]

Ideally the anesthesiologist should be called immediately to the emergency department to aid the trauma team. To examine an injured parturient, an initial 60-second comprehensive evaluation should be done.[4] If the patient is alert, one should get a brief history, which requires only a "yes" or "no" answer from the patient as one examines each region of the body and listens to the fetal heart sounds. The evaluation begins with observing the respiratory effort while one's hand is on the patient's radial pulse. If there is any sign of upper airway obstruction, clear the airway and intubate the trachea when indicated, and give oxygen. If tachypnea, tracheal deviation, rib fracture, or uneven chest expansion (possible hemothorax or pneumothorax) is indicated by palpation, draw arterial blood gases and aid in inserting a chest tube, if indicated. Gently palpate the cervical, thoracic, and lumbar spines, abdomen, pelvis, and the extremities for tenderness and fractures. Chest x-rays should be obtained when the patient is stabilized or in the operating room if required preoperatively.

If the patient responds inappropriately to simple questioning for orientation in time, person, and location, consider central nervous system injury or hypoxia due to shock.

Auscultation after palpation of the chest for the breath and heart sounds for detection of suspected hemothorax and pneumothorax and any concomitant disease is important in the anesthetic management. For a wheezing asthmatic patient ketamine as an induction agent is preferred to sodium pentothal, which may aggravate the bronchospasm.

Hemothorax, pneumothorax, cardiac tamponade, and hypovolemia are readily reversible causes of hypotension in a multiple trauma victim. In all injured parturients the supine hypotension syndrome must be recognized. It is due to pressure of the gravid uterus on the major vessels, namely, the inferior vena cava and abdominal aorta, leading to reduction of the venous blood return and cardiac output and interferes with the uterine blood supply. As a rule, any parturient of 16 weeks of gestational age or more should be placed with left uterine displacement by placing a wedge under the right hip. In an injured and hypovolemic parturient the supine hypotension syndrome is exaggerated and can have a lethal outcome if unrecognized.

The presence of known or suspected cardiovascular diseases, such as mitral and aortic valve diseases, mitral valve prolapse, or any congenital abnormalities including coarction of the aorta, tetralogy of Fallot and Eisenmenger's syndrome, or severe anemia, will alter the anesthetic management plan.

Classification of patients (infra vitae) according to their physical status at the time of examination is essential for determining the anesthetic choice. For parturients a particular anesthetic technique may offer specific advantages. For example, regional anesthesia is preferred for minor injuries to the limbs. On the other hand, general anesthesia is preferred for severe trauma or trauma involving the trunk or head and neck. Whenever general anesthesia is chosen a state of full stomach must be considered. Thus, a rapid-sequence induction must be the technique of choice to facilitate endotracheal intubation even if the surgical procedure is a minor one. The rapid-sequence induction technique comprises rapid induction with intravenous induction agents followed immediately by suxamethonium to facilitate muscle relaxation, cricoid pressure (Sellick's maneuver)[5] to block reflux of gastric contents, laryngoscopy, and tracheal intubation with a cuffed tube and inflation of the tube cuff. The purpose of this is to prevent pulmonary aspiration of possible regurgitated gastric contents.

In the third trimester or in any parturient after 34 weeks of gestation, the patient should be considered to have a full stomach. Antacids such as sodium citrate or magnesium aluminum hydroxide should be given before induction of anesthesia either orally, if the patient's condition allows, or through a preexisting nasogastric tube.[6]

CLASSIFICATION OF PATIENTS

Class I

Patients in class I are those who sustained minor trauma with minimum blood loss or those having been resuscitated with fluid therapy, and surgical intervention is not an urgent necessity. Surgery can be deferred until a thorough preanesthetic evaluation and laboratory workup have been completed. In fact, surgery and anesthesia may be carried out for class I patients as an elective procedure.

Class II

Patients in class II have sustained a moderate degree of blood loss with vital signs within normal limits. The vital signs remain stable through the reflex compensatory mechanisms involving principally increased sympathetic vasomotor tone with resultant reduction in the venous capacitance and increase in venous return to the heart. These compensatory mechanisms may mask hypotension due to hypovolemia and cause dangerous hypotension during induction of anesthesia as a result of vasodilation.

Surgery for these patients, although frequent is not of an immediate life-saving nature. Thus, time is usually available to perform clinical, radiologic, biochemical, and hematologic evaluations and simultaneously to correct deficiencies, such as restoration of circulating blood volume by fluids or blood transfusion or chest tube insertion in case of pneumothorax, to optimize the patient's condition, and to elevate the patient to class I status. Then, anesthesia is administered accordingly.

Class III

Patients in class III require immediate surgical intervention as a life saving measure. Such severely traumatized patients are frequently thrust upon the anesthesiologist with minimum data available concerning previous medical history and physiologic status. Thus, one may have to accept all of the risks involved in the management of such patients.

If the fetus is not affected by the trauma and it is decided to continue the gestation process, intraoperative fetal heart rate monitoring may be of value if the surgical field is away from the monitoring area. The value of observing not only the direct and indirect effects of anesthesia on the fetus, but also the effects of surgical manipulations and pressure effects of retractors directly on the uterus and indirectly on the blood vessels which may interfere with the placental circulation, producing signs of fetal distress.

EFFECTS OF ANESTHESIA ON THE EMBRYO AND FETUS

Direct Effects

The effect of anesthetics and their metabolites on cellular growth and division have been shown by many studies. For example, exposure to halothane in concentrations of 0.7% or higher for 12 hours has been shown to interfere with the synthesis of DNA,[7] and a variety of anesthetics (infra vitae) can affect cell division.

Fetal death occurs in animals after exposure to anesthetics and toxic metabolites.[8] It is a dose related effect. Fetal vulnerability to anesthetic exposure is related to the stage of fetal development. The period of organogenesis is between 15 and 56 days of gestation in humans. Particular sensitivity of the central nervous system occurs during the period of myelination at a slightly later time. Factors affecting the myelin formation could produce irreversible sequelae.

The effect of different individual anesthetics is as follows.

Nitrous Oxide Many independent studies have shown that there is a significant effect on fetal growth, skeletal development, and death rate in both pregnant rats and incubating chicks exposed to concentrations from 50% to 80% of nitrous oxide for periods extending from hours to days.[9]

Halothane Exposure of pregnant rats to halothane (0.8%) for 12 hours has increased the incidence of anomalous skeletal development and fetal death.[10]

Methoxyflurane An increased death rate and anomalies occurred in chick embryos exposed to methoxyflurane concentrations of 0.5% and higher on third and fourth days. An increased fluoride content of fetal bone of the rats exposed to 0.2% of methoxyflurane for 4 to 20 hours. This occurs only if the exposure happens after the period of active ossification of fetal skeleton, which begins the 12th day of gestation.[11]

Enflurane No evidence of mutagenicity after exposure to enflurane has been demonstrated by different studies.

Human effects Schnider and Webster in 1965[12] found that anesthesia and surgery during pregnancy were associated with 15.6% incidence of low-birth-weight babies (2500 g) compared with 9.9% incidence in the control group. Premature labor appears to be related more to the surgical disease rather than to the anesthetic agent or any specific technique.[13]

Indirect Effects

The integrity of uteroplacental circulation and the maintenance of adequate placental perfusion pressure is vital for fetal well being. Any cause that reduces the placental perfusion, such as increased uterine activity or maternal hypotension due to any reason, may result in fetal hypoxia. The use of drugs such as methoxamine to treat hypotension or ketamine (1.1 mg/kg) to induced anesthesia is not recommended as they may increase the uterine tone.[14]

The effect of hyperventilation on the circulation is twofold, namely, mechanical and biochemical. Hyperventilation with a ventilator may elevate the mean intrathoracic pressure and thus reduce venous return to the heart, or hypocapnia produces vasoconstriction of the umbilical vessels. Furthermore hypocapnia also produces a shift of the maternal oxyhemoglobin dissociation curve to the left. This favors oxygen binding to the hemoglobin rather than releasing it to the fetus.[15]

Higher concentrations of oxygen should be given to the mother during surgery under either general or regional anesthesia. It has not been shown that maternal hyperoxemia at 1 atm can produce retrolental fibroplasia or premature closure of the ductus arteriosus in utero. However, for caesarean section hyperoxygenation of the other is not recommended as it was shown by Rorke et al in 1968[16] that low scores were associated with concentrations of maternal inspired oxygen above 50%.

Maternal pain and apprehension and the use of vasopressors have a deleterious effect on uterine blood flow and thus deterioration of fetal condition.

SPECIAL CONSIDERATIONS FOR CONCOMITANT DISEASES OR CONDITIONS

Diabetes Mellitus

The reported incidence of diabetes mellitus is 1 in 325 to 350 pregnancies the United States. It is a significant cause of maternal morbidity and a major cause of perinatal illness and death.

If a traumatized parturient is known to be a diabetic, several blood glucose determinations should be performed intraoperatively. If the patient is insulin dependent, small doses of regular insulin (5 to 10 U) are to be given intravenously during surgery. Regular insulin is preferred to other insulin preparations as it minimizes difficulties in the management during the immediate postoperative and the postpartum periods, when the insulin requirement declines rapidly.[14]

Dextrose in the intravenous fluids should be given with caution and should not be used before a scheduled caesarean section, as the newborn of such a mother has hyperinsulinemia which will produce neonatal hypoglycemia. Knepp[17] demonstrated that the administration of 1000-mL solutions containing 5% dextrose to normal mothers undergoing caesarean sections raises maternal blood glucose to 245 mg/mL in comparison to a normal value from a control group receiving 1000 mL of physiologic saline.

The fetus of a severely diabetic mother is considered in distress and may be severely depleted in compensatory reserves. It may not tolerate an additional insult such as hypotension resulting from maternal hypovolemia.

Congenital or Acquired Heart Diseases

Congenital or acquired cardiovascular disease will place the parturient at a particularly high risk because of its association with an increase in maternal mortality.

Each parturient with cardiac disease has individualized limitations of the cardiac reserve. Thus, each reacts differently to the physiologic changes in the cardiovascular system due to pregnancy. Invasive hemodynamic monitoring with a pulmonary arterial pressure hemodilution catheter offers insight into ventricular functions in the presence of increased cardiac output and work and blood volume. It also provides clear therapeutic aims and the opportunity to observe the responses to manipulation of various circulatory parameters such as preload and after load with their relationship to cardiac output.

Rheumatic valvular diseases are the major cardiac diseases in the child bearing age. Among them, mitral stenosis is the most common lesion (75% to 90%). The aims for a successful anesthetic management for mitral stenosis are described below.

1. Rapid ventricular rates may not be well tolerated. A rate above 100 beats per minute may dramatically decrease cardiac output, leading to pulmonary hypertension and pulmonary edema. Thus, tachycardia-producing drugs such as atropine, scopolamine, meperidine, ketamine, and pancuronium should be avoided.

2. Rapid intravenous fluid infusion without hemodynamic monitoring should be avoided. It may induce right-sided heart failure, pulmonary hypertension, pulmonary edema, or arterial fibrillation.

3. Rapid reduction in systemic vascular resistance without hemodynamic monitoring is risky. It will reduce venous return and cardiac output and induce compensatory tachycardia and its sequelae.

4. Hyperventilation or hypoventilation which leads to hypocarbia or hypercarbia should be avoided. The former produces pulmonary vascular constriction leading to pulmonary edema and its sequelae. The latter induces acidemia leading to reduced cardiac output and tachycardia.

In mitral or aortic insufficiency one must avoid bradycardia. Monitored reduction in systemic vascular resistance is recommended to reduce regurgitation. The heart rate should be maintained between 80 and 100 beats per minute. In aortic stenosis reduction in systemic vascular resistance in the presence of a fixed cardiac output will cause severe reduction in perfusion pressure to the hypertrophic myocardium and other vital organs.

Congenital heart disease, presents not only the problems of myocardial hypertrophy but also those of either a left-to-right, right-to-left, or bidirectional shunt. Any decrease in systemic vascular resistance or increase in right-to-left shunt will result in hypoxemia, tachycardia and peripheral cyanosis.

In parturients with cardiovascular disease monitoring should include a peripheral arterial catheter for instantaneous blood pressure measurement and sampling for blood gas determinations, a pulmonary arterial catheter with or without the option of cardiac output measurement for assessment of left ventricular function and cardiac output, and calculation of systemic vascular resistance. The invasive hemodynamic monitoring serves as an excellent guide for maintaining a proper balance between myocardial oxygen supply and demand.

Thermal Burns

Descriptions of management of burns in parturients are scarce in the medical literature. The largest series of 24 patients were reported by Zhang et al.[18] The data from them and others indicate that the fate of both mother and fetus is related to the percentage of body surface area burned and the degree of burn rather than to the gestational age. If the burned area of second and third degree is less than 20%, the outcome is good for both the mother and the fetus. If the area is 20% to 35%, the outcome is good for the mother, but premature labor or intrauterine fetal death can almost be expected. If the burned area of second and third degree is more than 35% the outcome is poor for both the mother and fetus. In spite of this recent data, two patients with third-degree burns involving 65% to 75% of the body surface area in early pregnancy survived with good healing and delivery of live birth newborns at term.[19,20]

Premature labor in parturients with thermal burns was attributed to the efflux of prostaglandins from the injured skin and the accumulation of lipoproteins, which are prostaglandin precursors that are smooth muscle stimulators, leading to contraction of the uterus and expulsion of the fetus.[21,22]

If surgical treatment is chosen for the parturient with a thermal burn, general anesthesia through a endotracheal cuffed tracheal tube is the method of choice. Suxamethonium should be avoided because it induces hyperkalemia resulting in cardiac dysrhythmias and even death. Nondepolarizing muscle relaxants, such as d-tubocurarine or pancuronium, could be used. Gallamine should be used cautiously, if at all, because renal insufficiency is a common occurence in burns.

Successful anesthetic management depends largely on the consideration of the multiple system effects of burns. These effects are as follows. 1) Reduction in cardiac output due to reduction in blood volume and the circulating myocardial depressant factor, which has been shown to exist in humans and experimental animals. 2) Generalized increased capillary permeability. This change in pulmonary capillaries may lead to severe congestion and pulmonary edema. 3) Hemoconcentration due to fluid loss to the extravascular compartment. 4) Hypermetabolic state which may simulate a thryoid storm. The metabolic rate may be doubled or tripled according to the degree of burn. 5) Decreased pulmonary functions. The functional residual capacity and both pulmonary and chest wall compliance are decreased. The minute ventilation will increase markedly reaching values as high as 40 L per minute. 6) Reduced renal functions due to decreased plasma volume and increased secretions of antidiuretic hormone. 7) Restrictive forces from circumferential burns. It can cause severe respiratory impaired dynamics.

Toxemia Of Pregnancy

Symptoms of preeclampsia rarely become manifest before the 24th week of gestation, except in the case of hydatiform mole. Although the etiology is unknown, it is thought to be related to decreased placental perfusion, resulting in excessive production of the vasoactive substances. The clinical triad of hypertension, proteinuria, and generalized edema is diagnostic and is frequently accompanied with hyperreflexia. Being a multiple-organ disease its major effects are on the cardiovascular system. The generalized vasoconstriction results in diminution of the intravascular volume to various degrees. This change makes the patient very vulnerable to any blood loss or any vasodilation induced by anesthetic drugs or any other cause. The input and output of fluids should be monitored carefully by central venous and indwelling urinary catheters.

Patients with preeclampsia have coagulopathy due to decreased fibrinogen levels and platelet counts and increased fibrin split products. Therefore, caution must be exercised with conduction anesthesia, inserting monitoring catheters, or performing tracheal intubation to avoid any additional complications to the gravity of the situation.[1,2,14]

REFERENCES

1. Aboulish E: *Pain Control in Obstetrics*. Philadelphia, JB Lippincott Co, 1977.
2. Bonica JJ: *Principles and Practice of Obstetric Analgesia and Anesthesia*, vol 1. Philadelphia, FA David Co, 1967, 1969.
3. Bonica JJ: Maternal physiologic alterations. *Obstet Analgesia and Anesthesia*. Berlin, Heidelberg, Springer-Verlag, 1972, p 1–24.
4. Price DP, Skalar DP: The multiply injured patient. *Res Staff Phys* December 1981;27:73–87.
5. Sellick BA: Cricoid pressure to control regurgitation of stomach contents during induction of anesthesia. *Lancet* 1961;2:404.
6. Roberts RB, Shirley MA: Reducing the risk of acid aspiration during caesarean section. *Anesth Analg* 1974;53:859.
7. Jackson SJ: The metabolic effect of halothane on mammalian hepatoma cells in vitro, inhibitions of DNA synthesis. *Anesthesiology* 1973;39:405.
8. Smith BE: Teratogenicity of inhalation anesthetics. *Progr Anesth*. Amsterdam, Excerpta Medica Foundation, 1970, p 319–323.
9. Fink BR, et al: Terotogenic activity of nitrous oxide. *Nature* 1967;214:146.

10. Bussard OA, et al: Fetal changes in hamsters anesthesized with nitrous oxide and halothane. *Anesthesiology* 1974;41:275.
11. Fiserova-Bergerova V: Fluoride in bone of rats anesthesized during gestation with enflurane, or methoxyflurane. *Anesthesiology* 1976; 45:483.
12. Schnider SM, Webster GM: Maternal and fetal hazards of surgery during pregnancy. *Am J Obstet Gynecol* 1965;92:891.
13. Smith BE: Fetal prognosis after anesthesia during gestation. *Anesth Analg* 1963;42:521.
14. James FM, Wheeler AS: *Obstetric Anesthesia and the Complicated Patient*. Philadelphia, FA Davis Co, 1982.
15. Moya F, Morishima HO, Schnider SM, et al: Influence of maternal hyperventilation on the newborn infant. *Am J Obstet Gynecol* 1965;91:76.
16. Rorke MJ, Davey DA, DuToit HJ: Fetal oxygenation during caesarean section. *Anesthesia* 1968;23:585.
17. Knepp N: Effects on newborn of hydration with glucose in patients undergoing C-section with regional anesthesia. *Lancet* 1980;1:645.
18. Zhang Y, et al: Burns during pregnancy: Analysis of 24 cases. *Chin Med J (Engl)* 1981;2:123.
19. Anson H: Stage severe burns in the pregnant patient. *Obstet Gynecol* 1973;L,2:259.
20. Schmitz JT: Pregnant patients with burns. *Am J Obstet Gynecol* 1971;110:57.
21. Anggard E, Jonsson CE: Efflux prostaglandins in lymph from scalded tissues. *Acta Physiol Scand* 1971;81:440.
22. Mulla N: Labor following severe thermal burns. *Am J Obstet Gynecol* 1958;76:1338.

CHAPTER 9

POSTOPERATIVE CARE

GEORGE W. MACHIEDO

As high-speed highway travel and interpersonal violence increase in our society, the number and severity of injuries increase proportionally. Pregnant women share much of the same risk factors as other segments of society, and so the number of seriously injured pregnant women treated in our emergency departments and surgical intensive care units should be expected to increase.

The initial management of the pregnant trauma patient has been discussed elsewhere in this book. This chapter will concentrate upon the problems experienced in the surgical intensive care unit, after initial stabilization and operative management of the injuries has taken place. Special emphasis will be placed on techniques of monitoring organ function, particularly cardiac and pulmonary functions. Current concepts of treatment of various organ failure syndromes will also be covered. Attempts will be made to point out differences between normal cardiac and pulmonary physiology and that seen during pregnancy.

Since the major cause of fetal mortality after trauma is maternal mortality[1] and since little if anything can be done directly for the fetus after trauma, this chapter will concentrate on the monitoring and treatment of the mother.

GENERAL PRINCIPLES OF INTENSIVE CARE MONITORING

Before discussing the specific techniques of critical care monitoring, it is important to understand some basic general principles. The first of these is that the patient should not be ignored while the numbers are interpreted. Although much of this chapter will be devoted to describing techniques for the acquisition of numerical data concerning the pathophysiologic status of the pregnant trauma patient and the interpretation of those data, it should be kept always in mind that the data are meant to supplement good clinical physical examination of the patient, not replace it. If the data generated disagree with the clinical observation of the patient, a very careful search for technical and/or mathematical errors in data collection should be carried out, particularly if major changes in the management of the patient are contemplated as a result.

Stemming from the first general principle is the second, that the nurse in the surgical intensive care unit belongs at the patient's bedside, not in front of a central nursing station monitor with its sophisticated computer. As opposed to cardiac care units, where detection of arrythmias is a major component of care, I feel that there is little if any need for central station monitoring in surgical intensive care units.

Computers are extremely helpful in doing the numerous time-consuming calculations needed to generate hemodynamics data and also to trend an individual patient's performance over time. However, there is very little data to support the use of a computer as a monitoring device in trauma patients. It has been shown that computers do not decrease the number of nursing personnel needed in an intensive care unit, and, again, I feel much more comfortable with a trained, caring, thinking nurse at the bedside.

With these somewhat philosophical considerations in mind, I will proceed with the evaluation and treatment of individual organ systems in the traumatized pregnant woman.

CARDIAC PATHOPHYSIOLOGY AND MONITORING

The overall function of the cardiopulmonary system is directed toward adequate delivery of oxygen to the tissue. As such the heart and lungs must be considered as a functional unit. However, in many cases their evaluation can be done initially on an individual basis.

The evaluation of the cardiac system has classically been limited to serial measurement of the pulse rate and arterial blood pressure. These parameters, particularly the pulse rate, still have great clinical significance. However, with the development of the flow-directed pulmonary artery catheter by Swan and Ganz and their subsequent development of thermodilution cardiac output determinations, it is now possible to obtain a much more objective evaluation of cardiac performance. This is done by obtaining a direct measurement of cardiac output and by measuring, calculating or estimating the four primary determinants of cardiac output, namely, heart rate, preload, afterload, and contractility.

SWAN-GANZ CATHETERIZATION

The techniques of introduction of the Swan-Ganz catheter have been well documented in numerous articles[2-4] and need not be repeated here. Of greater importance is the decision of when and in whom the catheter needs to be placed. It is clear that pulmonary artery catheters need not be placed in all, or even in a majority, of patients suffering serious trauma, whether or not they are pregnant. In a review of my own experience, I found that less than 15% of severe trauma patients required Swan-Ganz insertion, even though the majority of them were in shock upon admission. The critical point is to decide as early as possible that a patient needs invasive hemodynamic monitoring and then proceed with catheter insertion, rather than waiting until the patient has deteriorated to a point where it is too late to alter the pathophysiologic derangements. Criteria for Swan-Ganz insertion are listed in Table 9-1. As with any other procedure in medicine, there are risks associated with pulmonary artery pressure monitoring. These are listed in Table 9-2. The majority of these complications are technical in nature and can often be avoided by a strict adherence to protocol.

Table 9-1
Criteria for Swan-Ganz Insertion

1. Hemodynamic instability unresponsive to fluid challenge
2. History of previous cardiac disease (acute myocardial infarction, etc) in a patient at risk for hemodynamic instability
3. Preoperative evaluation for major surgery
4. Necessity to use positive end expiratory pressure at levels greater than 10 cm H_2O

Table 9-2
Complications of Swan-Ganz Catheter

1. Pneumothorax
2. Laceration of subclavian artery or vein
3. Catheter-related sepsis
4. Intracardiac knotting
5. Disruption of pulmonary artery
6. Endocarditis
7. Cardiac arrythmia
8. Pulmonary infarction
9. Subclavian vein/superior vena cava thrombosis

Just as a decision to insert a Swan-Ganz catheter should be made early, so should the decision to remove or change the catheter be undertaken as soon as is practical. Some authors suggest that the incidence of sepsis related to the pulmonary artery catheter increases sharply after the third day post insertion. It has been suggested that, if the need for hemodynamic data persists after 72 hours,[5] the original catheter be removed and a new one should be inserted. The majority of trauma patients should be stable enough after 72 hours that the information provided by the Swan-Ganz catheter is no longer essential.

CARDIAC OUTPUT

The ability to measure cardiac output at the bedside in an accurate, reproducible way by an easy-to-master, noncumbersome technique has revolutionized hemodynamic monitoring. The importance of the ability to measure cardiac output rests not only in knowing the value itself, but also because cardiac output is necessary to calculate some of the important derived hemodynamic parameters, such as systemic and pulmonary vascular resistances and left ventricular stroke work. These derived data can often provide more crucial information than the cardiac output itself.

Cardiac output in the normal adult ranges from 5.0 to 6.0 L/min. When expressed as a cardiac index, ie, divided by body surface area, normal is 2.5 to 3.5 L/m^2. Low cardiac outputs (below 4 L/min) are due to hypovolemia or cardiac failure. Occasionally, a septic patient will have a low cardiac output. However, this is almost always due to a functional hypovolemia secondary to peripheral pooling of fluid in dilated capacitance vessels or fluid sequestration in the area of inflammation (eg, peritonitis). These patients will respond with a normal or high cardiac output when the effective fluid volume is restored.

Increases in cardiac output above normal are more difficult to evaluate. The pregnant woman has a normal cardiac output which rises at a note of about 1.0 to 1.5 L/min to reach about 6 L/min at 10 weeks, with a small rise to about 7 L/min at 24 weeks which continues to term. This must obviously be kept in mind when evaluating the hemodynamic status of the pregnant trauma patient. Other causes of an elevated cardiac output are sepsis, postoperative or post-traumatic hypermetabolic state, anemia thyrotoxicosis, cirrhosis of the liver, and major arterio-venous fistulae.

As mentioned above, it is just as important to evaluate the four determinants of cardiac output as it is to measure cardiac output itself.

PRELOAD

Preload refers, in a physiologic sense, to the amount of stretch applied to a myocardial fiber just before its next contraction. The greater the stretch, up to a given point, the greater will be the force of contraction, all other factors being equal. The stretch of the myocardial fibers in vivo is determined by the left ventricular end diastolic volume. Since this is a difficult parameter to measure clinically, it has been assumed that left ventricular end diastolic pressure is directly and somewhat linearly related to the end diastolic volume. Since at the end of diastole, in the absence of mitral stenosis, there is no pressure gradient from the left ventricle, through the left atrium and pulmonary veins back to the pulmonary capillaries, left ventricular end diastolic volume is clinically monitored by the pulmonary capillary wedge pressure.

Normal wedge pressures are between 5 and 15 mmHg. They tend to be somewhat higher during pregnancy. It is extremely important, however, to avoid the idea of setting the wedge pressure at a "normal" level when attempting to restore hemodynamic stability. Rather, the wedge pressure should be kept as low as possible, consistent with adequate peripheral perfusion. The adequacy of peripheral perfusion can be ascertained by using the criteria in Table 9-3.

If these criteria return to normal, fluid infusion can be cut back to maintenance levels plus the replacement of ongoing losses. If, however, prefusion parameters do not return to nor-

Table 9-3
Criteria for Adequacy of Peripheral Perfusion*

1. Heart rate	Below 100
2. Extremities	Warm
3. Urine output	More than 30 mL per hour
4. Cardiac output	Greater than 6 L/min
5. Systemic vascular resistance	Less than 1200 dyne-sec-cm^5
6. Mixed venous PO_2	More than 35 mmHg
7. Arteriovenous oxygen difference	Less than 5 volumes %
8. Lactic acid	Less than 2 mg %

*It is important to remember that no one of these criteria is an absolute guarantee of adequacy of perfusion. Rather, it is the overall evaluation of these parameters that is of clinical value.

mal, the preload should continue to be increased until the upper limit of normal, approximately 15 mmHg, is achieved. At this point, an estimation of myocardial contractility must be made. Techniques for making this estimate are discussed below.

AFTERLOAD

Afterload is defined physiologically as the impedance against which the ventricle must eject blood. It is a very complex concept, involving the viscosity of blood, the spatial characteristics of the ventricle, and the elasticity and cross-sectional area of the vascular tree into which the blood is being ejected. In clinical practice, however, afterload is considered to be equivalent to the systemic vascular resistance (SVR). This parameter is derived from the formula:

$$SVR = [(MAP - CVP)80]/CO$$

where MAP is the mean arterial pressure, CVP is the central venous pressure and CO is the cardiac output. The answer is expressed in dyne sec cm^{-5}, and normal is between 900 and 1200. A value above 1200 implies vasoconstriction. If a patient has clinical evidence of hypovolemia, then this is a normal compensatory phenomenon, and therapy should consist of fluid administration. If, however, fluid volume is adequate and cardiac index remains low in the face of an elevated systemic vascular resistance, then judicious use of an afterload reducing agent such as nitroprusside is indicated. When using potent vasodilators to decrease afterload, it is essential that arterial pressure be monitored continuously with an indwelling catheter. Blood pressure can drop precipitously to levels that will impair myocardial blood flow and oxygen delivery, possibly to levels low enough to cause cardiac arrest.

CONTRACTILITY

Contractility is the inherent ability of the myocardial fibers to shorten at a given preload and afterload. There is no clinically available technique of measuring contractility directly or of calculating it from other measured parameters. We must therefore make inferences about contractility. This is done by constructing a ventricular function curve. The standard curve is demonstrated in Figure 9-1. In a normally contractile heart, as the preload (pulmonary capillary wedge pressure) increases, left ventricular function (cardiac output or left ventricular stroke work) should also increase, up to a point. This is demonstrated by curve ABC. If, however, a rise in pulmonary capillary wedge pressure does not increase the left ventricular stroke work (curve ABD), then this implies a defect in myocardial contractility. Treatment at this point should include the addition of a positive

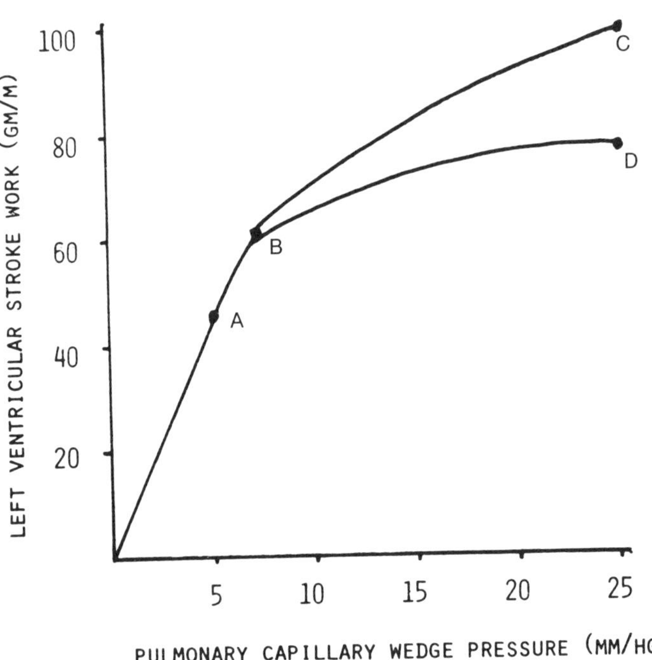

Figure 9-1 Ventricular function curve.

inotropic drug, such as dobutamine or dopamine, to improve the force of contraction and shift the curve up and to the left.

RESPIRATORY MONITORING

The primary aims of the respiratory system are to insure adequacy of oxygenation of arterial blood and to provide for removal of carbon dioxide from venous blood. These two functions can be monitored somewhat separately since in most trauma patients removal of CO_2 is ventilation dependent and not gas exchange dependent.

OXYGENATION

The ability of the lungs to adequately oxygenate arterial blood is classically ascertained by measuring the partial pressure of O_2 dissolved in plasma (PaO_2). However, in the critically ill patient following trauma, the measurement of PaO_2 alone is inadequate. Since many of these patients are on mechanical ventilators with additional oxygen added, the arterial PaO_2 can actually be misleading. A PaO_2 of 80 mmHg in a patient breathing room air would be acceptable, whereas the same PaO_2 in a patient on 50% oxygen would be indicative of a severe defect in oxygenation. For this reason, additional tests of gas exchange such as shunt calculation or alveolar-arterial oxygen difference are necessary to quantify the problem.

The transpulmonary shunt is the fraction of total cardiac output that goes past alveoli that have no ventilation and in which, therefore, no gas exchange takes place. Normally, the adult lung has a calculated shunt of below 5%. However, in the critically ill patient, this value frequently increases to 15% simply due to atelectasis, and if adult respiratory distress syndrome develops, then the shunt fraction can go as high as 40% to 50%.

Shunt is calculated by measuring (or calculating) the oxygen content of arterial blood and of mixed venous blood obtained from the distal lumen (pulmonary artery) of the Swan-Ganz catheter.

REFERENCES

1. Delancy JJ: Obstetrical and gynecological injuries in Zuidema GD, Rutherford RB, Ballenger WF (eds): *The Management of Trauma*. Philadelphia, The WB Saunders Co, 1979, p 483.
2. Swan WJC, Ganz W, Forrester Jr, et al: Catherization of the heart in man with the use of a flow directed balloon-tipped catheter. *N Engl J Med* 1970;283:447.
3. Civetla JM, Gabel JC: Flow-directed pulmonary artery caterization in surgical patients. Indications and modification of technic. *Ann Surg* 1972;176:753.
4. Cerra F, Milch R, Lajos TZ: Pulmonary artery catherization in critically ill surgical patients. *Ann Surg* 1973;177:37.
5. Sampliner JE, Pitluk HC: Hemodynamic and respiratory monitoring, in Berk JL, Samopliner JE (eds): *Handbook of Critical Care*. Boston, Little, Brown and Co, 1982, p 65.

CHAPTER 10

NEONATAL ASPECTS OF THE INJURED FETUS

NICOLE COHEN-ADDAD

GENERAL PERSPECTIVES

The occurrence of injury to the fetus is dependent upon the degree of protection provided by the mother-to-be.

Maternal Protection

In the dyad pregnant woman-fetus, the mother provides the enveloping material which protects the infant. The protection is effected through the amniotic fluid, the uterine wall, and the pelvis. This explains the higher degree of protection in the first trimester when the amount of amniotic fluid is proportionately greater,[1] and the uterus is still nested within the pelvis. The fetus is also better able to tolerate periods of maternal hypotension in early pregnancy than later on in gestation.[2] Thus, in the first trimester, although penetrating objects may produce fetal injury, blunt trauma is very unlikely to do so. No first-trimester abortion has yet been proven to be the result of trauma.[3] On the other hand, blunt trauma to the fetus, as well as trauma by a penetrating instrument, have been described in the second and third trimester; thus there are relative increases in incidence of fetal damage with increasing gestational age. However, since the first trimester is the time of organogenesis, chemical and radiation injuries are more likely to affect the fetus then rather than during organ maturation (second trimester) or nutritional storage (third trimester).

Incidence of Fetal Injury

The variety in types of injuries to the pregnant woman combined with the variability in their timing across gestation leads to a plurality of unique situations for the fetus. It is therefore, difficult to establish a general figure of the incidence of fetal injury resulting from trauma to the mother. About 25% of Americans are injured annually as a result of accidents. The accident rate during pregnancy has been reported in one study to be 6.9%.[4] Accidents were the most important cause of nonobstetric maternal deaths in the state of Minnesota from 1954 to 1964.[5] Although some figures are available for the pregnant woman, the incidence of fetal injury is not known. The latter has been the object of anecdotal case reports, but few comprehensive reviews have been published on the subject.[6-8]

Fetal Mortality

In the event of a trauma to the pregnant woman, maternal death represents the leading cause of fetal death.[9] Fetal survival is greatly compromised after 5 minutes from the time of maternal death to delivery.[10] When the mother survives, the most frequent cause of fetal death is placental separation.[9] Prematurity is an important cause of neonatal death secondary to injury in pregnancy. In a review of gunshot injuries, Browns et al recorded the mortality to be 78% for premature infants and 40% for term infants.[11]

VARIOUS CAUSES OF INJURY AND THEIR EFFECTS ON THE FETUS

The diversity in fetal damage is directly related to the diversity in causative mechanisms of injury to the pregnant woman. Since the management of the fetus is dependent on this plurality, it is essential to understand the cause-effect relationship between maternal trauma and fetal injury to anticipate the modalities of action regarding the fetus.

Maternal Traumas With Direct Effects on the Fetus

Blunt traumas represent 80% of all abdominal traumas in civil life[12] and are the result of automobile accidents in 50 to 85% of the cases.[10] Their diagnosis is often delayed in the presence of severe extra-abdominal injuries. However, their effects on the fetus can be devastating. Damage to the fetus can occur either by direct transmitted effect or by contrecoup mechanism against a fixed structure, most commonly the maternal sacral promontory.[13] The location of fetal injury is dependent on the fetal position at the time of maternal trauma. The head is the most frequently involved fetal part. In all six cases of intrauterine death with an intact uterus reported by Theurer and Kaiser, the fetal injury was localized to the head.[8]

Gunshot wounds to the pregnant uterus are more frequent than stab wounds. Since 1912, there has been no report of maternal death from gunshot wounds. However, the fetal outcome is still reserved. Buchsbaum reports 71% fetal deaths, some of which were due to prematurity.[10] Out of 73 reported cases in one review, 26 infants sustained substantial injuries with a mortality of 88%.[13] The other 47 survived with minor injuries to the extremities and soft tissues. The extent of the fetal injury depends on the trajectory of the bullet through the fetal tissue. While Wray et al[14] described a relatively benign case with only anemia, which corrected by itself, in Browns et al's case[11] the damage to the fetus was extensive with perirenal hematoma, laceration of the liver surface, perforation of the large bowels, and tension pneumothorax, notwithstanding prematurity (36 weeks). An exceptional case has been described by Buchsbaum and Caruso about a missile entering the fetus near the left nostril and producing no further damage, with subsequent deglutition and bowel elimination.[15]

Stab wounds to the abdomen of the pregnant woman have resulted from various penetrating pointed instruments, such as knives, files, pitchforks, scythes, sickles, and animal horns.[10] The maternal mortality from such wounds ranges from 3% to

10%. Fetal survival is very poor before 28 weeks of gestation. If the injury occurs later on in pregnancy, the fetus has a 50% chance of survival.

Because of the penetrating action, damage to the fetus can occur at any time in gestation, from curettage abortions induced by a variety of utensils to self-inflicted stab wounds at term.[16] Ocular perforation has been described during amniocentesis.[17] Intrauterine transfusions carry similar hazards, although with ultrasonography these procedures can be performed in a much safer way. The combined hazards of a certain type of instrument producing a wound at a certain time in gestation while the fetus is in a certain position does not allow for a systematized classification of this kind of wound. The fortuity of the situation is clearly reflected in Amine's case, where an 8-month pregnant woman stabbed with a barbecue fork delivered, a week later, a newborn with two small perispinal scars and "flappy legs" with flaccid paraplegia confined at 7 months of age.[18]

The effects of ionizing radiation in the first weeks of pregnancy have been described and studied extensively. The most susceptible organs are the brain and the eye with anencephaly, microcephaly, anophthalmia, microphthalmia, cataracts, colobomas, and retinal dystrophy. The critical radiation for teratogenicity to these organs is around 50 rads. This may be reached during diagnostic radiologic procedures. A dose of 100 rads is teratogenic to all fetal organs whereas a 260-rad accumulated dose may lead to abortion until the 14th week of gestation. The damaging effects of ionizing radiations are not limited to the first trimester, however. They can occur throughout gestation.

A case of fetal injury due to radiation therapy in late fetal life (at 30 and 33 weeks) has been reported by Gustavson et al.[19] The newborn was delivered at 36 weeks by caesarean section after failed induction to a woman with carcinoma of the uterine cervix who received irradiation to the pelvic area, including the fetal head, six and three weeks before delivery. There were no prenatal or postnatal asphyxia visible congenital defects at birth.

However, serial neurologic examinations in the next few months revealed progressive spasticity with myoclonic seizures and flexion contractures, and, later on, microcephaly with severe mental retardation. The ophthalmologic examination, initially normal, revealed on follow-up bilateral cataracts and microphthalmia.

Radiation during intrauterine life, even in low dose, multiplies the risks of leukemia in childhood by 1.5 and the risks of malignant central nervous system tumors by 10. It increases the percentage of spontaneous mutations. Moreover, there is no direct evidence that nonlethal radiation damage to the ovum can be repaired, although some studies suggest that there are no prior reasons for nonrepair of the human germ cells.

Certain chemicals ingested by the mother may cross the placenta and interfere with the fetus's own biochemical equilibrium. A few reviews have been published on the subject.[20–22] The action of the compounds on the fetus may be dependent on the timing of administration during gestation, from teratogenicity in the first trimester to intrauterine growth retardation in late gestation.

Iatrogenic direct trauma to the fetus during maternal surgery is probably a rarity. From a review of the literature, Buchsbaum has concluded that "laparotomy presents only minimal risks to the patient and the pregnancy."[10] One case report illustrates this resistance of the fetus under abdominal surgical manipulation. A surgical repair of a knife-induced perforation of the pregnant uterus was performed and a normal newborn was delivered three months later.[23]

Maternal Traumas With Indirect Effects on the Fetus

Injuries to organs in close connection with the fetus

Cord injury Cord lacerations by stab wound[24] or by bullet[25] with fetal bleeding into the amniotic fluid have been reported. Rarely, blunt trauma may result in rupture of an umbilical vessel.[26]

Placental injury Damage to the placenta is also seen more frequently after penetrating injury than blunt trauma, although both have been described. Placental laceration with hemorrhage leads to fetal anemia. In small placental separation (less than 25%), the threat to the fetus consists usually in premature birth with or without anemia. When more than 50% of the placenta is involved, fetal death is frequent.

Uterine injury Several cases of uterine rupture with prolonged in utero survival of the intact fetus have been reported.[27] However, uterine hemorrhage may represent a serious risk for the fetus's survival.

Rupture of the membranes Membrane tears after blunt trauma may lead to an important leak of amniotic fluid with production of oligohydramnios, which can mechanically prevent movement and expansion of the fetus, especially its lungs and extremities. But most often, the tears seal and the fetus develops normally.

Systemic internal injuries Fetal asphyxia may occur as a result of maternal hemorrhage, prolonged supine position, or stress related to the trauma. A common denominator to these situations is a decrease in uterine blood flow. In maternal hemorrhage, this represents an effort to maintain or restore the systemic blood pressure. In the case of prolonged supine position, the pregnant uterus compresses the aorta. During stress associated with trauma, the released cathecholamines produce a generalized systemic vasoconstriction with marked reduction in uterine blood flow. It has also been suggested that psychological trauma may precipitate a premature termination of pregnancy. Asphyxia to the mother also leads to fetal asphyxia, whether it is due to severe trauma to the lungs, central nervous system or to smoke inhalation. Rapid correction of the maternal asphyxia and good nursing care with adequate nutritional intake can save the fetus.[28]

Burns during pregnancy may affect the fetus in several ways. Fetal asphyxia may result from maternal shock in the most severe burn cases, whereas premature labor occurs usually within one week postburn[29,30] and may be due to presence of prostaglandin E_2 in the lymphatic fluid.[31] Thus, burn injuries to the pregnant woman can result in fetal distress and prematurity with possible fetal demise.

Unusual causes of injury have been described with actual or potential damage to the fetus. Envenomation of a pregnant woman by box-jellyfish has been reported, with delivery of a healthy full-term newborn nine weeks later.[32] The authors recorded on admission a maternal heart rate of 150/min with a blood pressure of 150/90. It is conceivable that the maternal tachycardia with normal blood pressure represented a compensatory cardiac action for a preshock situation with decreased uterine blood flow. A case of electric shock without loss of consciousness or permanent injury to the mother has led to the death of an otherwise normal fetus.[33]

Another trauma with little consequence to the mother, but harmful to the fetus, has been demonstrated in experimental conditions in the fetal sheep.[34] Acute decompression sickness was produced in fetuses exposed to deep dives for various periods of time. Massive air emboli were detected in the fetal, but not the maternal, circulation. At lower depths, the amount of air bubbles decreased accordingly. Although it is unlikely that a pregnant woman would risk herself and her fetus in a deep dive consciously, except in a case of suicidal attempt, the risk may be real in the early gestation of a sport-oriented mother not yet aware of her pregnancy.

DIAGNOSIS OF INJURY TO THE FETUS

The in utero assessment of the fetus can be performed at the time of the accident or shortly afterwards. The disappearance of fetal movements witnessed by the mother is very suggestive of fetal death. When abdominal x-rays are needed for the management of the mother, the film may incidently reveal a fracture of the fetal limbs[35] or skull. It also may help localize a missile or shrapnel. The monitoring of the fetal heart rate is a general indication of fetal death. Poor or absent beat-to-beat variability in the absence of maternal drug intake or fetal tachycardia in the third trimester can be an ominous sign of fetal distress. Severe tachycardia or bradycardia hold a reserved prognosis. Fetal death is suspected when fetal heart rate cannot be recorded. Ultrasonography has recently enlarged our scope of vision regarding the fetus. It allows for the diagnosis of limbs, spine, or skull fracture and confirms the location of a missile or other objects. Nonradiopaque material such as wood can also be detected. Uterine perforation with a wooden stake has been described.[10] Real time ultrasonography may suggest a fetal demise by the absence of fetal breathing or more general fetal movements. Amniocentesis may reveal the presence of blood in the amniotic cavity, possibly a sign of fetal hemorrhage. Perforation of the fetal bowel, when suspected from the location of a missile or other instrument inside the fetal abdomen, may be diagnosed by amniography, which reveals the presence of radiopaque dye in the fetal peritoneal cavity.

The postnatal assessment of the injured fetus consists of a general evaluation and a systemic study of each organ.

General Examination

The general examination focuses on the search for signs of prematurity, asphyxia, anemia, infection, and gross congenital anomalies.

The gestational assessment by Dubovitz or Ballard scoring is essential to establish the fetus's viability and to project a plan of action for future management of the preterm infant. In prematurity, the mortality is mostly related to lung immaturity, and intracranial hemorrhages account for most of the morbidity. Asphyxia is suspected in the presence of apnea, bradycardia, cyanosis, and poor peripheral pulses.

Anemia is often difficult to determine by clinical observation at the initial physical examination since asphyxia itself may produce pallor through the diving reflex phenomenon. As in all mammals, diving and asphyxia lead to a redistribution of the blood away from the periphery toward the vital organs. In asphyxia pallidum, the normovolemic nonanemic infant has extreme pallor through this mechanism. On the other end, anemia with hypovolemia is suspected with a history of heavy maternal bleeding around the time of delivery and the persistently poor femoral pulses even after correction of asphyxia. Anemia with normovolemia or hypovolemia is suggested when the physical examination of the newborn reveals signs of compensatory efforts like tachycardia or hepatosplenomegaly, sometimes associated with generalized edema. In Wray's case, anemia was the only fetal injury occurring after extensive maternal abdominal gunshot wounds.[14]

Infection is suspected by history of the type of injury, and clinically in the presence of vasomotor disturbances with sudden changes in color and peripheral perfusion or, more rarely, when purulent lesions of the soft tissues are discovered.

Gross congenital anomalies, such as anencephaly, anophthalmia or other teratogenic malformations are easily recognized. More subtle abnormalities such as imperforate anus, cleft palate, etc need to be investigated.

Assessment of Organ Systems

A step-by-step assessment of the newborn by organ systems in the nursery follows the initial general evaluation done in the delivery room.

Clinically, the head is inspected for asymmetry, deformed head shape, and ecchymoses. The palpation may outline a fracture of the skull as reviewed by Alexander and Davis[13] or a cephalhematoma. The jaw may be fractured.[36] The examination of the eyes may reveal posttraumatic damage by a pointed instrument, anophthalmia or microphthalmia from intrauterine exposure to radiations, asymmetry of the pupils size and light reflex from intracranial compression or damage of the third cranial nerve or an asymmetric doll's eyes sign from injury to any of the oculomotor nerves.

The neck palpation may reveal a crepitus of the clavicles. Fractures of the clavicles are frequently seen after injury in utero.[7]

The chest is inspected for asymmetry. Its palpation may discover the presence of rib fractures. Absent breath sounds on auscultation suggest the possibility of a pneumothorax or a diaphragmatic hernia of teratogenic or traumatic origin. In Browns' case, both a pneumothorax and a traumatic diaphragmatic hernia were produced in the fetus by a maternal thoracoabdominal gunshot wound.[11] Postasphyxial tricuspid insufficiency is frequent and will manifest as a soft transient heart murmur above the xyphoid.

The abdomen is an important part of the newborn's examination, especially in the presence of anemia, since hemorrhage can extend freely into the peritoneal or retroperitoneal cavity. Subcapsular hematoma or liver laceration have resulted from intrauterine injury.[11,37] An enlarged and tensed liver (more than 3 cm below the right costal margin) may be present, with or without hemorrhage into the peritoneal cavity. Renal and perirenal hemorrhage can occur too.[11,37] An enlarged mass may be palpated. Traumatic perforation of the bowel may be totally asymptomatic. However, any sign of abdominal rigidity, tenderness, distension, and paraumbilical blueness of the skin is very significant. A scaphoid abdomen suggest a diaphragmatic hernia.

The extremities are examined for the presence of ecchymoses and deformities and palpated in search of a mobile fracture or a callus. Uhde reported in 1856[38] the presence of callus formation at the level of the clavicle and humerus in a term infant born 2 months after maternal injury. Fetal fractures of the legs, arms, and scapula—by a pitchfork— have resulted from intrauterine trauma.[7,35]

Involvement of the fetal spine is rare. Fracture and dislocations of the cervical spine[36] and spinal cord lesion—with a barbecue fork[20]—are anecdotal. However, in the face of a trauma to the pregnant uterus, they need to be ruled out. On physical examination, a superficial lesion may be present around the spine. A decrease in tone and reflexes of the extremities may be present at birth.

Soft tissue involvement may be self-limited or represent a point in the trajectory of the offending instrument. It may be minimal as in the case described by Buchsbaum and Caruso[15] wherein the portal of entry of the missile was missed on initial examination since it was narrow and covered with vernix. More extended lesions have been reported such as the superficial lacerations seen on the fetus's back and left flank after intrauterine trauma with a kitchen knife.[16] In the nursery, seizures and decerebrate posturing from intracranial hemorrhage may develop.

Blood gas determinations are done to evaluate the extent of the asphyxia and/or pulmonary insufficiency. The hematocrit reflects the level of anemia. The white cell count may suggest an infectious process. The presence of hematuria suggests renal damage, either traumatic or postasphyxial. The superficial cultures evaluate the presence of a colonization, whereas blood and spinal cultures may reveal septicemia and/or meningitis.

Transillumination of the chest is positive in the presence of a pneumothorax. The chest x-rays may confirm the diagnosis or reveal a diaphragmatic hernia. The film may also discover rib or clavicle fractures. Abdominal obstructive series can demonstrate the presence of fluid in the peritoneal or retroperitoneal cavity, possibly a bleed. Levels of fluid in the lumen of the bowels suggest intestinal obstruction. A pneumoperitoneum may be the reflection of bowel perforation. x-rays of the extremities will confirm a fracture suspected clinically. Vertebral fractures are rarely suspected clinically. They often represent an incidental finding in chest x-rays. However, in the face of a violent trauma to the fetus, they need to be searched for.

The real-time ultrasonography of the head can delineate subependymal, intraventricular, and intraparenchymal hemorrhages.

The computerized tomography scan adds information in regard to the subdural and subarachnoid spaces and helps suggest a contusion process in the presence of intracerebral hypodense areas. However, in previously reported cases of intrauterine head injury, before the era of ultrasound echography and computerized scanning, the intracranial hemorrhages were mostly diagnosed at the time of autopsy.[39-42] It is interesting to note that intracranial hemorrhage can occur without skull fracture, as a result of intrauterine injury.[24]

Ultrasound of the abdomen may confirm an enlarged kidney containing blood, a subcapsular hematoma, or a pneumoperitoneum.

MANAGEMENT OF THE INJURED FETUS

In utero, the correction of maternal hypotension and the prevention of infection will favorably influence the fetal outcome. The reestablishment of a good uterine blood flow is essential for the survival of the fetus and its normal intrauterine growth. Abdominal trauma to the mother does not necessarily signify immediate delivery of the fetus. Unless maternal hemorrhage, infection, or interference in the exchange between mother and fetus is present, the removal of the preterm fetus is unwarranted, due to the potential severe complications associated with prematurity. Even a ruptured uterus can be repaired leaving the fetus in utero.[10]

Postnatally, the asphyxia, which is primarily respiratory in origin, is best treated with 100% oxygen and bag-valve-mask or endotracheal ventilation. Atropine may reverse the diving reflex. Epinephrine will correct the bradycardia. Bicarbonate is used sparingly since its adminstration in premature infants has been associated with an increased incidence of intracranial hemorrhages. Trishydroxyaminomethane is a preferred buffer in newborn resuscitation since it decreases pCO_2 unlike bicarbonate. In case of untractable bradycardia, an isoproterenol (Isuprel) drip is started. A dopamine drip is used only after previous slow infusions of volume expanders have been given. These are administered only when a maternal history of heavy bleeding around the delivery time is associated with poor or absent femoral pulses in the neonate, since their administration has also been associated with an increased incidence of intracranial hemorrhages, especially in the sick premature infant whose absence of blood pressure autoregulation allows for transmission of rapid pressure changes to the cerebral vessels.

The anemia, usually acute, requires urgent correction, preferably with O-negative, unmatched whole blood infused slowly. If the anemia is not severe, typed and cross-matched blood will be administered. When the hemorrhagic trauma has occurred several days to weeks before delivery, a fetal compensatory mechanism may have restored its blood volume. In such cases, the pallor, the suggestion of past intrauterine trauma, and a hematocrit value may be the only elements of information, although generalized edema may be present. When this presentation is suspected, a central venous pressure determination through an umbilical vein catheter will confirm the normovolemic or hypervolemic state of the patient. A plasmapheresis, with replacement of the removed blood by packed red cells, is then indicated.

Infections related to intrauterine trauma caused by organisms already present in the amniotic fluid or the placenta such as Group B *Streptococcus* and *Escherichia coli* infections are treated with penicillin or ampicillin and gentamycin. When contamination by organisms carried on the offending object itself is suspected, ampicillin and clindamycin are preferred. Tetanus coverage depends upon previous maternal immunization status and treatment. When needed, human serum antitoxin alone is given to the neonate. The metabolic disorders secondary to prematurity, intrauterine growth retardation or asphyxia, are corrected by glucose or calcium infusion.

The respiratory therapy includes thoracentesis in case of pneumothorax and oxygen supplementation with or without ventillatory support in the presence of idiopathic respiratory distress syndrome secondary to prematurity.

Seizures due to asphyxia, intracranial hemorrhage, or central nervous system contusion are treated with phenobarbital, alone or in combination with phenytoin when necessary.

Surgical procedures include general surgery of the abdomen, chest, and soft tissues to stop a hemorrhage, to remove an object, to repair a laceration or perforation of an organ, or to debride a superficial lesion. Continuous or intermittent nasogastric suctioning and stabilization of the infant's vital signs and metabolic equilibrium (fluid, electrolytes, glucose, calcium, and blood gases) are preferable when possible before the surgery.

Orthopedic consultation does not necessarily imply surgery. Fractures of the clavicles or the extremities will often heal without manipulation or surgery. The osteoblastic activity of the infant usually allows for a good healing process without deformities.

Neurosurgical intervention is required mainly in the view of a subdural hemorrhage with symptomatology or a severely depressed skull fracture.

PROGNOSIS

Prematurity carries the risk of intracranial hemorrhage with the possibility of progressive hydrocephalus and mental retardation. The immature eyes may develop retrolental fibroplasia. The lungs may become dependent on oxygen supplementation and develop bronchopulmonary dysplasia. The intestines are very sensitive to hypoxia, and necrotizing enterocolitis may present by 1 to 3 weeks of life. The ductus arteriosus is patent and often symptomatic, especially at 4 to 5 days of age when the pulmonary vascular resistance diminishes. The premature infant, initially on ventilatory support for hyaline membrane disease, then requires support for pulmonary edema in relation to the ductus arteriosus.

The postasphyxial syndrome includes signs of renal failure with hematuria and oliguria or polyuria by acute tubular necrosis. Transient tricuspid insufficiency may be present.

Hypoglycemia, hypocalcemia, and hypomagnesia are frequently seen. Seizures may develop, usually after 12 hours of life. Their characteristics are varied.[42] Subtle seizures are seen in both preterm and term infants. They range from fluttering of the eyelids with horizontal deviation of the eyes to oral-buccal-lingual movements and rowing or pedaling of the extremities. Generalized tonic seizures are characteristic of the premature infant, especially with intraventricular hemorrhage. Multifocal clonic seizures are seen more often in the full-term neonate.

Of all the organs, trauma to the head carried the most reserved prognosis, with the possiblity of central nervous system damage. Chest lesions are usually limited and respond well to treatment. Abdominal lesions can be fatal if the hemorrhage is uncontrolled, but when the bleeding is limited, the prognosis is usually good. Injuries to the spine bear various outcomes according to the degree of involvement of the spinal cord and the level of the lesion.

Although most lesions due to intrauterine injury will be visible or symptomatic at birth, radiation damage in later pregnancy can stay undiagnosed for months. Such maternal history may therefore require an extended follow-up of the infant.

CONCLUSION

Although the embryo seems protected against blunt trauma during the first trimester of pregnancy, most other modalities of injury avail in all gestational periods. The variety of agents lead to a diversity in fetal involvement. Aside from fetal demise, the neonatal morbidity is essentially governed by asphyxia, anemia, prematurity, and central nervous system complications.

REFERENCES

1. Gadd RL: The volume of the liquor ammi in normal and abnormal pregnancies. *J Obstet Gynecol Br Commonw* 1966;73:11.
2. Buschbaum HJ: Splenic rupture in pregnancy. Report of a case and review of the literature. *Obstet Gynec Surg* 1967;22:381.

3. Javert CT: Role of the patient's activities in the occurence of spontaneous abortion. *Fertil Steril* 1960;11:550.
4. Peckham CH, King RW: A study of intercurrent conditions observed during pregnancy. *Am J Obstet Gynecol* 1963;87:609.
5. Hakanson EY: Trauma to the female genitalia. *J Lancet* 1966; 86:287.
6. Brinton JH: Report of two cases of intrauterine fracture, with remarks on this condition and references to 51 cases already reported by different writers. *Trans Am Surg Assoc* 1884;2:425.
7. Smith RR: Intrauterine fracture: Report of a case and review of the literature. *Surg Gynecol Obstet* 1913;17:346.
8. Theurer DE, Kasier IH: Traumatic fetal death witout uterine injury: Report of a case. *Obstet Gynecol* 1963;21:477.
9. Crosby WM, Costiloe JP: Safety of lap belt restraint for pregnant victims of automobile collisions. *N Engl J Med* 1971;284:632.
10. Buchsbaum HJ: Accidental injury complicating pregnancy. *Am J Obstet Gynecol* 1968;102:752.
11. Browns SK, Bhat R, Jonasson O, et al: Thoraco-abdominal gunshot wound with survival of a 36-week fetus. *JAMA* 1977;237:2409.
12. Allen RB, Curry GJ: Abdominal trauma: A study of 297 consecutive cases. *Am J Surg* 1957;93:398.
13. Alexander E Jr, Davis CH Jr: Intrauterine fracture of the infant's skull. *J Neurosurg* 1969;30:446.
14. Wray RC Jr, Burnett WF: Gunshot wound of the intestine, pregnant uterus, and placenta with maternal and fetal survival. *Am Surg* 1971;37:308.
15. Buchsbaum HJ, Caruso PA: Gunshot wound of the pregnant uterus. Case report of fetal injury, deglutition of missile, and survival. *Obstet Gynecol* 1969;15:425.
16. Knapp RC, Drucker DH: Self-inflicted stabwounds to pregnant uterus and fetus at term. *NY State J Med* 1972;72:391.
17. Oglesby R: Eye trauma in children. *Pediatr Ann* 1977;6:11.
18. Amine AR: Spinal cord injury in a fetus. *Surg Neurol* 1976;6:369.
19 Gustavson KH, Jagell S, Blomquist HF, et al: Microcephaly, mental retardation and chromosomal aberrations in a girl following radiation therapy during late fetal life. *Acta Radiol* 1981;20:209.
20. Adomson K, Joelsson I: The effects of pharmacological agents upon the fetus and newborn. *Am J Obstet Gynecol* 1966;96:437.
21. Dentkos, M: Passage of drugs across the placenta. *Am J Hosp Pharm* 1966; 23:139.
22. Mirkin B: Effects of drugs on the fetus and neonate. *Postgrad Med* 1970;47:91.
23. Badia PD, Charlton A: Stabwound of a seven-month pregnant uterus. *NY State J Med* 1940;40:1797.

24. Dyer I, Barclay DL: Accidental trauma complicating pregnancy and delivery. *Am J Obstet Gynecol* 1962;83:907.
25. Martins CP, Garcia OM: Ferimentos do utero gravido por arma de fogo. Revisao de literatura communicacao de um caso. *An Brasil Ginecol* 1964; 58:229.
26. Stowe HM: Rupture of the umbilical cord. *Am J Obstet* 1902; 46:792.
27. McNabney WK, Smith EI: Penetrating wounds of the gravid uterus. *J Trauma* 1972;12:1024.
28. Sampson MB, Peterson LP: Post-traumatic coma during pregnancy. *Obstet Gynecol* 1979;53:2S.
29. Schmitz JT: Pregnant patients with burns. *Am J Obstet Gynecol* 1971;110:57.
30. Yingbei Z, Xuewei W, Yingjie Z, et al: Burns during pregnancy. *Chin Med J [Engl]* 1981;94:123.
31. Anggard E, Jonsson CE: Efflux of prostaglandins in lymph from scalded tissue. *Acta Physiol Scand* 1971;81:440.
32. Williamson JA, Callanan BI, Hartwick RF: Serious envenomation by the Northern Australian box-jellyfish. (Chironex fleckeri). *Med J Aust* 1980;1:13.
33. Peppler RD, Labranche FJ Jr, Conneaux JJ: Intrauterine death of a fetus in a mother shocked by an electrical current: A case report. *J La State Med Soc* 1973;124:37.
34. Fife WP, Simmang C, Kitzman JV: Susceptibility of fetal sheep to acute decompression sickness. *Undersea Biomed Res* 1978;5:287.
35. Bucholz R, Mauldin D: Prenatal diagnosis of intrauterine fetal fracture. A case report. *J Bone Joint Surg* 1978;60:712.
36. Crosby WM: Trauma during pregnancy: Maternal and fetal injury. *Obstet Gynecol Surg* 1974;29:683.
37. Connor E and Curran J: In utero traumatic intra-abdominal deceleration injury to the fetus. A case report. *Am J Obstet Gynecol* 1976;125:567.
38. Uhde CWF: Beitrage geburtschulflichen inhalts, Part 2, Fractur der calvicula und des os humeri im mutterleibe. *Monatsschr Geburtsk* 1856;8:22.
39. Atlay RD, Prysor-Jones D: Blunt external abdominal trauma causing fetal death. *Am J Obstet Gynecol* 1967;97:577.
40. Watts CC, Clark K, McConnell TH: Fetal head trauma without maternal uterine injury. *Am J Obstet Gynecol* 1967;99:289.
41. Handel CK: Case report of uterine rupture after an automobile accident. *J Reprod Med* 1978;20:90.
42. Volpe JJ: Neonatal seizures—Part I, Differential. *Perinat Care* 1977;1:19.

CHAPTER 11

CHEST TRAUMA IN PREGNANCY

ALEXANDER F. ZOLLI
WILLIAM E. NEVILLE

Trauma still ranks as the chief cause of death in people up to 38 years of age, accounting for 164,000 deaths in 1980.[1] Furthermore, one-fourth of all accidental civilian deaths result from thoracic injury.[2] Bearing these statistics in mind, the risk of accidental injury to the gravid patient becomes readily apparent. Our modern society offers a variety of hazards to the pregnant woman. Automobile travel, "controlled" violence of athletic competition, and injury inflicted by knives and gunshot wounds set the scenario of accidents incurred during pregnancy. The overall incidence of accidental injury in the gravid patient stands fixed at 6% to 7% of all pregnancies.[3] A number of reports cite accidents as one of the common nonobstetric causes of death among pregnant women.[4-6]

The anatomic and physiologic changes that accompany pregnancy can alter the body's response to injury. Direct fetal injury notwithstanding, it is the interrelationship of maternal and fetal factors that forms the basis of the unique sequence of events after injury. A firm understanding of the basic cardiorespiratory features in the gravid state forms the cornerstone of logical and accurate care of thoracic injury during pregnancy. Therefore, we shall consider first some aspects of maternal and fetal physiology before reviewing specific chest injuries.

ANATOMIC AND PHYSIOLOGIC PRINCIPLES

Maternal Features

The maternal cardiovascular system adapts to the demands of the increased metabolic state by increasing the total blood volume 30% to 50%.[7,8] Plasma volume increases proportionately more than the red cell mass. This "physiologic anemia" of pregnancy may serve to confuse accurate assessment of blood volume, but during periods of stress, ie, shock, this hypervolemic state enhances maternal tolerance to hemorrhage. More specifically, it has been shown that the pregnant woman can maintain stable vital signs and adequate tissue perfusion during a 10% to 20% acute blood loss[9] and even up to 30% to 35% of a gradual blood loss.[10] Part of this hemostasis occurs at the expense of the fetus.

The heart undergoes an actual shift in position and apparent increase in the roentgenographic silhouette. The area of dullness is increased by virtue of the anterior rotation and left upward displacement. The apical impulse is displaced 1 to 1.5 cm beyond the maximal point in the normal nonpregnant woman. Physiologically, a soft systolic murmur is noted in more than 50% of pregnant patients, and extrasystoles are not uncommon. Both pulse rate and cardiac output are slightly increased.[8] In cases of mediastinal injury, these subtle anatomic and physiologic changes can pose diagnostic pitfalls to the unknowing observer.

The lining of the respiratory tract from the nasal mucosa to the terminal airways undergoes increased congestion and engorgement, a situation that can possibly lead to difficulty in breathing and/or retained secretions. Diaphragmatic excursion is not reduced, but a 4-cm elevation in the level of the diaphragm is apparent on chest x-ray examination. The anteroposterior and transverse diameters of the chest undergo expansion most marked as the bases of the hemithoraces. Total lung and vital capacities remain relatively unaffected, but the minute ventilation increases to 50% above normal. Important to the trauma setting is the fact that the gravid patient counteracts developing respiratory embarrassment by increasing her respiratory rate rather than the depth of tidal volume, admittedly a less efficient mechanism.[11]

Fetal Features

In the setting of maternal chest injury, fetal well being and survival is threatened by *direct* damage from penetrating thoracoabdominal trauma as well as by the *indirect* mechanisms of inertial forces (blunt trauma), hypoxia, and shock.

The gravid uterus is usually well protected by the pelvic framework during the first trimester. However, penetrating wounds of the lower chest can jeopardize fetal survival when the trajectory of the offending agent finds a path through the enlarged uterus of later pregnancy. Uterine, placental, umbilical cord, and fetal damage collectively or individually can result from wounds entering through the chest.

Blunt chest injury severe enough to rupture the amniotic sac and membranes can precipitate premature labor. Inertial forces and shock can cause premature placental separation with resultant partial or complete abruptio. In one report,[12] the finding of maternal shock carried an 80% fetal mortality. As stated above, the mother can tolerate states of hypovolemia rather well and for considerably longer periods of time than can the fetus. During stress and shock, maternal vital organ blood flow is enhanced at the expense of the fetus. The uterine arteries constrict, thereby reducing perfusion through intervillous spaces. The resultant hypoxia from impaired uterine blood flow severely tests fetal viability. Vasoconstrictors have little utility in the treatment of hemorrhage shock inasmuch as they may further increase fetal hypoxia via the mechanism of uterine arterial spasm. Moreover, reduced fetal oxygenation has also been demonstrated with severe material hyperventilation, as may occur in response to pain, anxiety, or respiratory insufficiency.[11] Prolonged hypoxia (anoxia) is universally fatal.

TREATMENT OF CHEST TRAUMA

Thoracic injuries in the pregnant woman should be managed the same as in the nonpregnant one. The pervading principle is that maternal well-being is paramount. Expeditious treatment of maternal injury to guarantee survival also offers the best chance for fetal survival. Patients with severe chest injury are frequently in a critical condition and in need of immediate care, but only about 15% of them ultimately undergo thoracotomy. The great majority of cases can be adequately treated by procedures that should be available in the emergency room (Table 11-1 and 11-2). The principal tasks in the initial resuscitation of the chest injured revolve around establishing a patent airway, stabilizing

Table 11-1
Suggested Emergency Room Protocol In Serious Chest Trauma to a Pregnant Woman

Rapid general assessment
Establish and maintain a patent airway
Support tissue perfusion (treat shock)
Chest x-ray
Electrocardiogram
Cross-matching of blood
Monitor adequacy of volume state (central venous pressure, Swan-Ganz lines
Correct hypoxia and/or acidosis
Insert nasogastric tube and urinary bladder catheter
Doppler monitoring of the fetus

Table 11-2
Vital Emergency Diagnostic and Therapeutic Modalities in Chest Injury

Tube thoracostomy	Aortography
Autotransfusion	Pericardiocentesis
Emergency thoracotomy	

a flail chest segment, relieving pneumohemothorax, controlling hemorrhage, and supporting circulation. It is assumed that the critical care of this unique patient will be rendered and shared by the total trauma team namely, the chest surgeon, traumatologist, intensivist, and obstetrician.

Generally Applicable Measures

Chest injury can seriously affect the normal ventilatory mechanism. The resultant hypoxia from diminished gas exchange poses the major threat to the mother. It is to be vigorously avoided both for her ultimate benefit and to preclude intrauterine catastrophe. Patient evaluation in this regard includes two points: 1) assessment of patency of the airway and 2) assessment of the adequacy of ventilation. Increased respiratory secretions normally attend pregnancy, and it is in the gravid patient that respiratory support in the form of endotracheal intubation or tracheostomy is frequently required. Insertion of a radial arterial line will allow ready access for serial blood gas determinations. This provides reliable data as to the adequacy of ventilation. In this way, specific acid-base imbalances can be identified immediately and corrected appropriately. Evacuation of gastric contents by passage of a Levine tube precludes the risk of accidental airway aspiration and also reduces the infradiaphragmatic pressure exerted by that viscus on the ipsilateral hemithorax.

Cardiovascular dynamics are readily supported by infusion of lactated Ringer's or saline solution via two large-bore central intravenous lines. Right atrial pressure or pulmonary capillary wedge pressure measurements by the respective central venous pressure and Swan-Ganz catheters allow accurate evaluation of the changing blood volume pattern. An indwelling urinary bladder catheter monitoring urinary output serves as an indirect check of tissue perfusion and alerts the trauma team to possible associated renal injury. Vasopressor agents are not recommended to support maternal blood pressure in the hypovolemic period because of the untoward effect on intrauterine circulation.

Thorough evaluation and care of the trauma victim is not complete until blood is sent to the laboratory for cross-match and typing, the electrocardiogram is run, and antibiotic and tetanus prophylaxis is administered. In the first instance, an available source of blood products is mandatory since ongoing blood loss can be indeterminate and demands appropriate volume repletion. Auto-transfusion, when possible, is the optimal modality to counteract acute blood loss in chest trauma. The electrocardiogram tracing supplies baseline information and indicates ST segment and T wave changes suggestive of myocardial contusion or ischemia. It also alerts the physician to life-threatening arrhythmias that can be quickly corrected. In general, once the pleural space has been violated by a penetrating injury, it becomes a contaminated space. Appropriate antibiotics and antitetanus coverage should be given to avert the late sequelae of empyema, sepsis, and tetany. Maternal sepsis is a leading cause of fetal mortality.

Fetal heart rate monitoring can be performed at the bedside via the non-invasive Doppler technique. This quick and convenient adjunct supplies vital information to the obstetrician and should be an available part of the diagnostic armamentarium in the emergency ward.

Normally, radiation exposure during pregnancy is kept to a strict minimum. However, roentgenographic examination of the chest is compulsory in every case of thoracic trauma. It remains the fundamental method of determining osseous and visceral injury. There must be no hesitation in obtaining the necessary views. Radiation exposure can be kept to a minimum by conventional shielding maneuvers and unnecessary studies and duplication of films must be avoided. Radiation exposure from computer-assisted tomography tends to be almost the same as that from conventional techniques, but reportedly produces less scatter. This modality has become a valuable diagnostic tool in the evaluation of thoracic problems and should be kept in mind for selected persons.

Fractures of the bony thorax not only represent the most common injury to the chest wall, but also account for the most prevalent cause of ventilatory impairment. The pain associated with rib fracture limits the depth of respiration, and the secondary muscular splinting involuntarily limits chest wall excursion. These two conditions result in impairment of ventilation. Isolated fractures of the ribs and clavicle are best managed conservatively. Analgesics form the mainstay of therapy. Taping of the chest is an outdated modality and bears mention here only to condemn its use. For multiple rib fractures, especially those located on the lower left chest and associated with significant pain and muscle splinting, hospital evaluation for 48 to 72 hours is advocated.

Tube thoracostomy is to the management of chest wounds what digitalis means to the treatment of the failing heart. Whether due to blunt or penetrating trauma, the majority of thoracic injuries are managed by the insertion of a chest tube. A hemothorax is promptly drained, and continued bleeding can be accurately assessed. When used for pneumothorax, the placement of a chest tube evacuates any air present, reexpands the atelectatic lung, and helps restore full ventilatory capacity. Three principles generally apply to the proper use of tube thoracostomy. First, a chest x-ray is not necessary before placement of a chest tube. In the severely injured patient, clinical signs of absent breath sounds, compromised cardiac performance, and shifted mediastinum mandate early employment of closed thoracostomy. Second, only large bore (32 to 40 Fr) and straight chest tubes should be inserted. Blood may clot in smaller chest tubes, precluding effective drainage whereas the use of right-angled tubes makes proper positioning difficult at best. Third, in the gravid patient, the chest tube should be inserted behind the pectoralis major muscle in the anterior axillary line and above the level of the nipple, since the diaphragmatic dome is elevated during pregnancy and normally reaches this height in full expiration.

Thoracotomy as supportive or definitive therapy in chest trauma may be employed in the emergency ward or is more commonly performed in the operating room suite after stabilization, evaluation, and preparation of the patient have been completed. Prompt thoracotomy should be performed in the emergency room when cardiac arrest occurs from either tamponade or hypovolemic shock. The rationale in the former case rests upon the fact that immediate pericardial decompression may be lifesaving. In the latter instance, open cardiac massage improves the resuscitative effort in the seriously hypovolemic person. The more conventional indications for thoracotomy are covered in the next section on specific injuries.

Specific Injuries

Injuries to the chest have long been arbitrarily defined as either blunt or penetrating. Recently, Lewis[2] subdivided the entire group into two categories: immediately life threatening and relatively life threatening (Table 11-3).

We should preface this discussion by stating that, in general, thoracotomy with or without pulmonary resection is consistent with the successful conduct of pregnancy. Moreover, there is too little risk attendant upon thoractomy to support the uncertainty of prolonged observation, particularly in the precarious gravid trauma patient.

Immediately life-threatening situations

Airway obstruction Foreign bodies, copious secretions, severe facial trauma, and laryngeal fracture commonly result in

Table 11-3
Blunt and Penetrating Chest Trauma

Immediately life threatening	*Relatively life threatening*
Airway obstruction	Penetrating great vessel injury
Open pneumothorax	Pulmonary contusion
Tension pneumothorax	Myocardial contusion
Flail chest	Diaphragmatic rupture
Massive hemothorax	Esophageal perforation
Cardiac tamponade	Tracheobronchial tree rupture
Air embolism	

acute obstruction to ventilation. The resultant asphyxia is fatal to both mother and fetus. Treatment, therefore, is aimed at establishing a dependable airway either by removing the responsible agent or, as stated previously, by intubation, tracheostomy, or cricothyroidotomy.

Open pneumothorax This open communication with the outside instantly collapses the underlying lung and prevents normal negative thoracic pressure mechanics. Respiratory distress is the immediate result. Treatment centers on two goals. First, an airtight cover must be placed over the defect. Next, tube thoracostomy is employed to evacuate the intrapleural air and reexpand the lung.

Tension pneumothorax Seepage of air into the pleural space without a means of escape as with a one-way valve mechanism has two grave consequences. Impaired ventilation from lung collapse and restricted venous return to the heart from contralateral mediastinal shifting can combine in a fatal outcome. Immediate tube thoracostomy is the definitive therapy.

Flail chest The impact of a blunt object against the thoracic cage can result in sternal or multiple rib fractures at multiple sites. This flail segment moves in a paradoxical motion compared with the uninvolved chest, ie, outward with expiration and inward with inspiration. The larger the flail portion, the more the respiratory dynamics are altered. Instability of the bony thorax prevents build-up of negative intrathoracic pressure, thereby nullifying the movement of air into and out of the trachea. This condition is commonly seen in automobile steering wheel accidents. Successful treatment is directed at stabilizing the chest wall. External fixation by turning the patient on the affected side or by other artificial devices may be difficult to maintain. Internal (pneumatic) fixation via intubation and mechanical positive pressure ventilation is generally the preferred means of therapy.

Massive hemothorax Continuous copious bleeding (more than 300 cc/hour) from the thorax after chest tube insertion usually heralds major vessel damage. Common sources of such hemorrhage are the pulmonary hilum, internal mammary and intercostal arteries, or the aorta itself. Autotransfusion here is a valuable measure in attempting to replete the blood volume rapidly. However, the burden of responsibility with continued massive blood loss rests upon prompt control of the bleeding site. Only timely surgical intervention will save this type of patient.

Cardiac tamponade The patient who is brought to the emergency room in shock and with distended neck veins after blunt or penetrating chest injury carries a diagnosis of acute cardiac tamponade until proven otherwise. The overall rate of survival depends not only on the treatment, but also on the nature and severity of the injury. Aspiration of the hemopericardium (pericardiocentesis) should be employed only as a diagnostic or initial therapeutic measure. It may be life-saving in some instances by the removal of only 20 to 30 mL of blood. However, prompt thoracotomy with suture repair of the source of bleeding is universally advocated. The injury can usually be repaired without the use of cardiopulmonary bypass. When the hemorrhage emanates from the surface of the heart, the surgeon must exercise great caution to avoid injury of the coronary arteries with the repair sutures. Using this method of prompt thoracotomy for suspected cardiac injury, Neville and Bolanowski[13] have reported improved survival from 14% to 58% in a series of 58 consecutive patients.

Air embolism This not uncommon injury can follow either penetrating or blunt trauma. A fistulous communication between the bronchial tree and the pulmonary venous system represents the basic pathophysiology. The sequelae of such an event may result in neurologic and myocardiac damage or death to both mother and fetus. Diagnosis is difficult at best. There are, however, three strongly suggestive clues. The finding of penetrating chest injury and focal neurologic deficits without obvious head injury should alert the observer to the possibility of air embolism. Cardiovascular collapse after intubation and a brief period of positive pressure ventilation is a second suspicious setting. Last, obtaining frothy blood-tinged sputum from the endotracheal tube or froth from an aspirated arterial line is evidence in support of this diagnosis. Unfortunately, despite appropriate therapy, this condition is not compatible with survival in every case.

Relatively life-threatening situations

Injury to the great vessels Major transection or a large traumatic rent of a great vessel is generally fatal within minutes. Approximately 15% of patients will survive long enough to reach the hospital because of incomplete rupture or a tamponading effect of nearby viscera. These patients remain at high risk since 90% of them undergo subsequent rupture within 48 hours after injury if untreated. In daily civilian trauma, this form of chest injury occurs commonly in deceleration auto accidents and in falls from significant heights. The patient's general status may vary from profound shock to borderline instability. Diagnostic suspicion is aroused when a massive amount of blood is returned from the tube thoracostomy or reviewing the chest films (Table 11-4). Aortography is very helpful both to delineate the exact site of injury and in planning the operative approach. The possible risk to the fetus from the angiographic procedure must be weighed against the ultimate catastrophe of double death from maternal exsanguination. Left thoractomy with interposition of a Dacron tubular graft and utilization of a Gott shunt is standard protocol for injuries distal to the left subclavian artery. Cardiopulmonary bypass with systemic

Table 11-4
Roentgenographic Indications for Angiography In Aortic Trauma

Mediastinal width greater than 8 cm (100 cm AP supine chest x-ray)
Tracheal shift to the right
Blurring of aortic outline
Obliteration of medial aspect of left lung (pleural capping)
Opacification of clear space between aorta and left pulmonary artery
Depression of left main stem bronchus below 40°

heparinization may be needed for aortic arch injuries. The attendant obstetrical risk of this latter approach must be borne in mind and demands the continued attendance of responsible personnel to monitor and treat any intrauterine reaction.

Pulmonary contusion Little has been written about parenchymal lung contusion, but it remains one of the more frequent injuries encountered in blunt thoracic trauma, with or without disruption of the bony thorax. The "bruising" of lung substance is followed by disruption of alveoli, bronchioles, and blood vessels with resultant intraparenchymal hematoma formation. The treatment is straightforward and includes reexpansion of the lung, maintenance of a patent airway, and ventilatory support when indicated.

Myocardial contusion This rarely fatal condition is likely misdiagnosed in many instances. It is commonly encountered with impact injury in the sternal area. The patient often experiences arrhythmias in the period immediately after injury. ST segment and T waves changes on the electrocardiogram suggestive of pericarditis or ischemia characterize myocardial contusion. Definitive diagnosis is offered by serial myocardial enzyme studies and nuclear scanning. This is generally a self-limiting problem and should be treated in context with any associated injury by bed rest and arrhythmia monitoring.

Diaphragmatic rupture After blunt injury or actual penetration, diaphragmatic rupture often remains an occult injury. It may have a symptom-free interval of viable length. Recently, two cases of delayed traumatic rupture of the diaphragm were detailed by Dudley et al.[14] Treatment is directed toward early surgical intervention. Acute rupture is best approached via laparotomy, whereas a thoracotomy is advocated in delayed conditions. Delivery of the infant should be deferred unless labor is imminent and onset of labor within four weeks of corrective surgery should probably be terminated by cesarean section before the onset of the second stage of labor.

Esophageal perforation This type of wound is almost always secondary to penetrating injury. Depending upon the actual level of disruption, symptoms will vary. Diagnosis should be suspected when the patient complains of pain and the x-ray films disclose cervical or mediastinal emphysema or pleural effusion. Hypaque esophageal swallow and esophagoscopy confirm the diagnosis. Contamination of the mediastinum and pleura by saline and gastric contents produces early chemical and later bacterial mediastinitis. If the injury is recognized within 24 hours, primary repair should be attempted. Cervical esophageal injury can be repaired primarily by direct suture and drained. Thoracic perforation demands exploration for repair and wide drainage. A high index of suspicion must be maintained here since failure to recognize and treat an esophageal disruption is commonly fatal. Moreover, the development of frank mediastinitis as a source of maternal sepsis can terminate in fetal death.

Tracheobronchial tree rupture The majority of patients who develop this condition will demonstrate some degree of pneumothorax, and all will show a pneumomediastinum on chest x-ray. Bronchoscopy is diagnostic. The mainstays of treatment are 1) establishing an airway beyond the point of the tear for adequate ventilatory effort, 2) insertion of a chest tube to evacuate any associated pneumothorax, and 3) thoracotomy for direct closure of the rent as the definitive step.

Complications

The initial resuscitation and treatment of the gravid thoracic patient may be lifesaving, but strict surveillance is necessary in the period after injury so as to detect any possible problems (Table 11-5). The incidence of these complications varies and is, in general, related to multiple factors. Yet it behooves the physician to monitor carefully, diagnose early, and treat aggressively, thereby allowing the pregnancy to continue safely. Apart from direct intrauterine damage, fetal well-being and survival is secondarily related to maternal death, sepsis, and shock.[3]

In the gravid patient, posttraumatic aspiration, atelectasis, pneumonia, and empyema either individually or in combination

Table 11-5
Chest Trauma Complications

Aspiration
Atelectasis
Pneumonia
Empyema
Respiratory failure (adult respiratory distress syndrome)
Myocardial (pump) failure

can lead to the development of maternal sepsis. The ultimate effect on the fetus is unpredictable, but several serious complications have been described, namely, fetal hypoxia, sepsis, and prematurity.

A prominent finding and often principal cause of late death after trauma is respiratory failure due to adult respiratory distress syndrome. The adult respiratory distress syndrome may be defined as respiratory insufficiency due to interstitial pulmonary edema without evident cardiogenic etiology. Its onset in the majority of trauma victims develops late, that is, from seven to 21 days after injury, and is most commonly associated with systemic or pulmonary sepsis. The incidence has been estimated at 6% in over 6,000 patients surveyed by Lewis et al.[15] The mortality associated with adult respiratory distress syndrome is significant, with a 38% figure cited after thoracic trauma.[16] Prompt control of sepsis is the most important factor determining outcome for both mother and fetus.

Immediate myocardial (pump) failure can result from numerous causes: tension pneumothorax, pericardial tamponade, myocardial contusion, myocardial infarction, and coronary air embolization. The direct consequence is maternal shock with impaired oxygen delivery to the peripheral organs. Fetal mortality has been listed as high as 80% after documented maternal shock. Immediate restoration of acceptable tissue perfusion by correcting the underlying condition offers the best chance of maternal and fetal salvage.

SUMMARY

Major thoracic trauma to the pregnant woman represents the challenge of managing two lives. Yet the interests of the fetus generally coincide with those of the mother so that pregnancy itself should not delay or compromise maternal therapy. In most cases, the mother's chest injury can be effectively treated without endangering the conduct of pregnancy. Understanding the gravid patient's altered response to trauma and the attendant risks imposed upon the unborn will help guarantee a favorable outcome. In essence, the approach to this unique patient should be borne by the combined effects of surgeon and obstetrician: maternal well-being insures the health of the fetus.

REFERENCES

1. Trunkey DD: Overview of trauma. *Surg Clin North Am* 1982;62:3.
2. Lewis FR: Thoracic trauma. *Surg Clin North Am* 1982;62:97.
3. Baker DP: Trauma in the pregnant patient. *Surg Clin North Am* 1982;62:275.
4. Baino A, Freeman DW, Baker MP Jr: Minnesota mortality study. *Minn Med* 1962;45:847.
5. Crosby WM: Trauma during pregnancy: Maternal and fetal injury. *Obstet Gynecol Surg* 1974;29:683.
6. Montgomery TA, Lewis A, Hammersly M: Maternal deaths in California, 1957–1962. *Calif Med* 1964;100:412.
7. Wilson JR, Beecham CT, Carrington ER: *Obstetrical and Gynecological Surgery* ed 5. St Louis, CV Mosby, 1975.
8. Kaminetzky HA, Iffy L: *Principles and Practice of Obstetrics and Perinatology*. New York, John Wiley & Sons, 1981.
9. Romney SL, Gavel PV, Takeda Y: Experimental hemorrhage in later pregnancy. *Am J Obstet Gynecol* 1963;84:636.
10. Dilts PV Jr, Binkman CT III, Kirschbaum TH, et al: Uterine and systemic hemodynamic interrelationships and their response to hypoxia. *Am J Obstet* 1969;103:133.
11. Bains MS, Beattie EJ Jr: Thoracic surgery in pregnancy, in Barber HRK, Graber EA (eds): *Surgical Diseases in Pregnancy*. Philadelphia, The WB Saunders Co, 1974.
12. Rothenberger D, Quattlebaum FW, Perry JF, et al: Blunt maternal trauma. A review of 103 cases. *J Trauma* 1978;18:173.

13. Neville WE, Bolanowski PJP: Cardiac trauma, in Goldsmith, H (ed): *The Practice of Surgery*. Hagerstown, Md, Goldsmith Publishers, 1981.
14. Dudley AG, Teaford H, Gatewood TS Jr: Delayed traumatic rupture of the diaphragm in pregnancy. *Obstet Gynecol Surg* 1979;53:255.
15. Lewis FR, Blaisdell FW, Schlobohm RM: Incidence and outcome of post-traumatic respiratory failure. *Arch Surg* 1977;112:436.
16. Olcott C, Barber RE, Blaisdell FW: Diagnosis and treatment of respiratory failure after civilian trauma. *Am J Surg* 1971;122:260.

CHAPTER 12

ORTHOPAEDIC TRAUMA AND THE PREGNANT PATIENT

IRVING G. STRAUCHLER

The automobile has become the major mode of transportation in America, and it has also become a major cause of orthopaedic trauma in America today. Similarly, the automobile is a major cause of orthopaedic trauma in the pregnant woman. The increased mobility afforded the pregnant woman has increased her exposure to serious trauma. In early studies of pelvic fractures, Noland and Cornwell[1] in 1930 found the incidence of pelvic fractures in women to be 50% of their series as contrasted to 10% reported in 1923.[2] In 1937, the percentage of women sustaining pelvic fractures rose to 60% in a series by Eliason and Johnson.[3]

There is a continuing trend for women to enter hazardous occupations formerly held solely by men. More and more women are working later into pregnancy than previously. Both of these facts have increased the exposure of pregnant women to occupational orthopaedic trauma.

OPEN FRACTURES

Open fractures are surgical emergencies. The basic management is unchanged in the pregnant woman, although management of a specific injury may require modification in pregnancy.

Open fracture wounds by definition are contaminated wounds and if left untreated will become infected wounds.

Gustillo[4] has classified open fractures into the following three types: type I, fracture with minimal contamination, a laceration 1 cm or less with minimal soft tissue damage; type II, same as type I, except laceration is larger than 1 cm; and type III, open fracture with extensive soft tissue crushing or damage.

The principles of open fractures include the following. 1) early adequate irrigation and debridement; 2) adequate and appropriate antibiotics; 3) fracture stabilization, either cast or external or internal fixation; 4) safe, appropriate wound coverage; and 5) early cancellous bone grafting.

Lower extremity venous pressure increases as pregnancy progresses. This increased venous pressure can produce increased bleeding from lower extremity fractures and lacerations. This in turn can predispose to compartment syndromes. Delayed wound closure is essential in most type II and all type III open fractures. Recent studies[4] have shown that cancellous bone grafting done early in the course of open fracture management has led to early fracture and wound healing.

Wound skin defects with a diameter less than 5 cm usually will close spontaneously without the need for complicated procedures, such as cross leg flaps, which would represent unusual difficulties in the pregnant patient.

VASCULAR INJURIES AND ORTHOPAEDIC TRAUMA

In the case of certain patterns of injury, vascular damage must be under high suspicion. Dislocation of the knee can damage the popliteal artery. Proximal tibia fractures can damage the trifurcation to the popliteal artery into its three divisions: the peroneal, anterior, and posterior tibial vessels. Dislocations of the elbow and supracondylar fractures of the humerus can affect the brachial artery. Doppler studies and digital subtraction arteriography should be preferred if possible to regular arteriography due to its attendent risks, especially in pregnancy.

UPPER EXTREMITY TRAUMA

Hand Injuries

Pregnancy as such has little specific impact on the management of common upper extremity injuries. During the second and third trimester, however, peripheral edema increases, affecting the hand and wrist region, and is often associated with carpal tunnel syndrome, which commonly occurs with pregnancy. Although there is no definite answer to the causal mechanism, the suggested theories include the following: 1) the effect of the hormone estrogen, 2) the increase in peripheral edema, and 3) soft tissue changes including flexor tendon synovial thickening.[5]

Minor trauma, which could be overlooked by the nonpregnant woman, may produce an acute carpal syndrome in the pregnant patient. Similarly fractures about the distal radius and ulna, the carpus, and hand may also bring on an acute carpal tunnel syndrome. Symptoms consist of numbness, tingling, and paresthesia in the radial three and one-half digits of the hand (the sensory distribution of the median nerve). Complaints of clumsiness and dropping of objects are frequent. A common early complaint is awakening at night with severe pain and paresthesia in the hand, which is relieved by shaking hand and wrist.

Carpal tunnel syndrome in pregnancy should be treated nonsurgically if at all possible. Most cases resolve postpartum; in fact, some patients experience relief while still on the delivery table! Therapy should include wrist splinting at night and diuretics if symptoms warrant. Steroid injections should be avoided. Postpartum, resistant cases can be treated with the usual surgical decompression. Where there is significant open wound about the area of the hand, wrist, and forearm, requiring surgical intervention, then surgical decompression of the carpal tunnel in the face of such trauma may be indicated during pregnancy.

Most hand surgery can be done under regional or local anesthesia. Most phalangeal fractures are stable with closed reduction and require only 2 to 3 weeks of immobilization. The care of unstable hand fractures may require surgery, and this should not be delayed awaiting delivery, due to the rapid onset of stiffness and malunion in this region. The results of repair of tendon lacerations similarly have been shown to be superior when done promptly Isolated digital nerve repairs may be delayed if the patient is several weeks from term. All unstable displaced intraarticular fractures should be promptly surgically corrected. Regional or local anesthesia presents little risk to the pregnant patient.

As women in the second and third trimester are more awkward, falls on the outstretched hand are expected to be more common. The Colles' fracture is the most common wrist fracture in adults, predisposing to the carpal tunnel syndrome as noted above. Accurate reducation is exceedingly important in the young adult. If accurate reduction cannot be maintained by closed means, then pin fixation above and below or open reduction with internal fixation may be indicated. Navicular fractures also occur with a fall onto the dorsiflexed wrist, and this injury may not appear on initial x-rays. With tenderness and pain in the "anatomical snuff-box," even in the face of normal x-rays, this injury should be treated with immobilization and x-rayed again after two weeks.

Forearm Trauma

Displaced fractures of both bones of the forearm in the adult are usually unstable and require open reduction and internal fixation. Cast immobilization may be used, and surgery may be delayed up to two weeks to allow delivery. Prolonged delay or inadequate reduction often leads to loss of pronation-supination motion.

Minimally displaced radial head fractures should be treated with splinting for symptomatic rest for one to two weeks followed by range of motion exercises.

Other interarticular elbow fractures with displacement require accurate reduction and usually require surgery.

Upper Arm and Shoulder Trauma

All dislocations require prompt reduction. Anterior dislocation of the shoulder accounts for 95% of all glenohumeral dislocations. The first episode of shoulder dislocation in the young adult requires four weeks of immobilization. This may be troublesome in late pregnancy, but is important. Various methods of immobilization such as the stockinette Velpo sling may allow more comfort in the pregnant patient.

Similarly, humeral shaft fractures present special problems in pregnancy. Most humeral shaft fractures can be treated with cast immobilization, either a hanging cast or coaptation splint (a double sugar tong). This type of care requires the patient to sleep in a semisitting position, to allow for the weight of the arm and plaster to maintain fracture alignment. The protuberant abdomen of late pregnancy may lead to fracture angulation. If the patient is nonambulatory, overhead or to the side skeletal traction may be needed to maintain alignment. These fractures usually heal rapidly and often after two weeks may be treated with an adjustable plastic cylinder cast brace, popularized by Sarmiento et al. This type of cast care allows for both elbow and shoulder motion while maintaining fracture alignment. This type of cast brace is least affected by the body habitus of pregnancy and should be preferred.

CERVICAL SPINE TRAUMA

Facial injuries and head contusions are commonly associated with fractures of the cervical spine. Any multiple trauma patient with such injuries must have full radiologic evaluation of the cervical spine done at the time of initial evaluation. This should include flexion and extension x-rays. Cervical contusions or hyperextension-hyperflexion injury without fracture or ligamentous instability of the cervical spine can be treated in the pregnant patient as in the general population with cervical collar, analgesics, and rest.

Most cervical spine fractures are stable and only require a cervical orthosis as well as symptomatic analgesics. Unstable cervical spine dislocations or fractures may be treated with a halo vest, which can be modified to accommodate the enlarging breast and abdomen in pregnancy. In clinically unstable cervical fractures, pregnancy should not affect the course of surgical management to prevent neurologic damage. Women with cervical spine instability are at significant risk of neurologic trauma during labor if not stabilized before that (Figure 12-1).

THORACOLUMBAR TRAUMA

The lordosis of pregnancy, increases in weight, the shifting of the center of gravity, and pendulous heavy breasts all predispose to lower and upper back pain with an increase in pressure on previously compromised nerve roots. Minor trauma can produce nerve compression with distal neurologic symptomatology.

As many of these factors resolve postpartum every effort should be made to treat pregnant patients with lower and upper back pain nonsurgically. In the face of trauma, the workup should include adequate x-rays with flexion and extension if necessary to delineate whether there is a fracture or a ligamentous injury that can cause instability of the spine. Recent chymopapain has been approved for use in the treatment of disk disease in the United States. The effects of chymopapain in pregnancy are as yet unknown.

Most fractures of the thoracolumbar spine are minor anterior wedge compression fractures. These require symptomatic treatment consisting of bed rest and analgesics. At times, a hyperextension brace is needed. These can be modified for the pregnant patient's growing abdomen.

Unstable fractures in this region require surgical stabilization, and the patient should not be allowed to go into labor without stabilization as further injury may result.

Devices such as the Roto-Rest bed have made the nursing care of patients with unstable spinal injuries much easier.

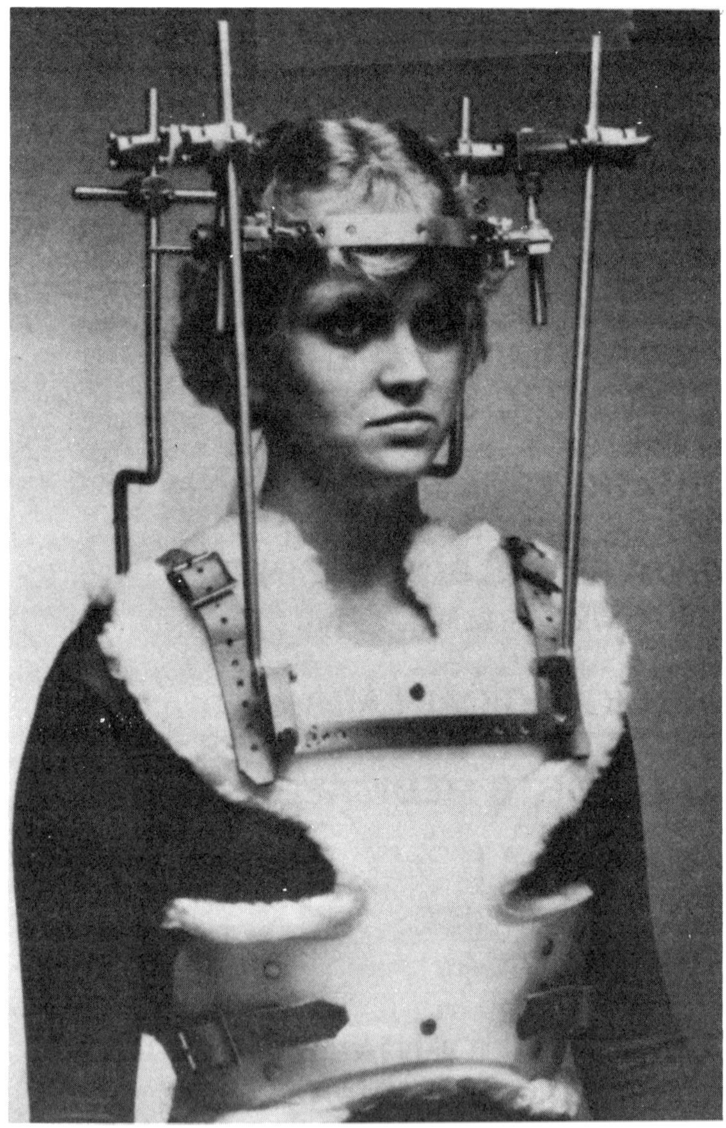

Figure 12-1 Twin-cities Lo-profile Halo system. (Courtesy of DePuy, Inc.)

Special attachments for the operating room table allow positioning of the patient prone with hip and knees flexed, relieving pressure on the abdomen, which is especially important in the pregnant patient (Figure 12-2).

SPONDYLOLISTHESIS

The forward subluxation in this condition of one vertebrae on the other, usually L5 on S1, may be asymptomatic. However,the weight increase and lordosis of pregnancy coinciding with trauma may lead to an acute increase in the amount of slip, leading to acute neurologic problems as well as interfering with the fetal inlet to the pelvis. The lithotomy position may worsen this situation, and caesarean section may be necessary.

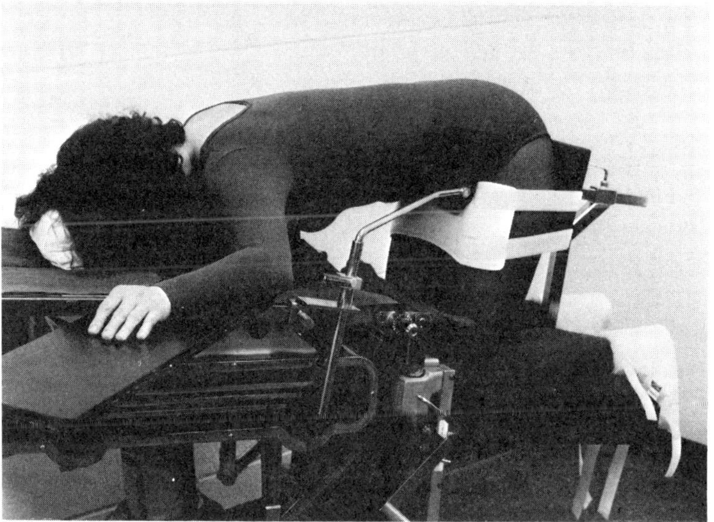

Figure 12-2 Andrews spinal surgery frame. (Courtesy of Orthopedic Systems, Inc.)

PELVIC FRACTURES

Pelvic fracture is the orthopedic injury of greatest concern to the obstetrician. A simple classification of fractures of the pelvis is outlined below: 1) minor avulsion fractures, 2) isolated rami fractures, 3) acetabular fractures, and 4) pelvic ring fractures.

Pelvic ring fractures have been classified by Tile, and Pennal et al[6] based on the direction of force as follows: 1) anteroposterior compression, 2) lateral compression (ipsilateral anterior and posterior lesion, contralateral anterior and posterior lesion [bucket-handle], four-rami and posterior lesion, and miscellaneous), and 3) vertical shear.

Patients with pelvic fractures must be assumed to have visceral injuries until proven otherwise. It is disastrous to focus one's attention on a large uterus and an obvious pelvic fracture and to ignore potentially fatal visceral injuries. McMurtry et al[7] reviewed associated injuries in 79 multiple trauma patients with pelvis fractures (Tables 12-1 and 12-2).

As can be seen from the above data, pelvic fracture occurring during pregnancy is associated with increased fetal loss and pelvic fracture occurring before pregnancy is associated with increased incidence of cesarean section.

Table 12-1
Injuries Associated with Pelvic Fractures (79 Cases)

	No. of Patients	Associated Mortality	Percent
Respiratory system	49	11	22
Cardiovascular system	5	2	40
Central nervous system	36	10	28
Gastrointestinal system	23	12	52
Genitourinary system	10	2	20
Musculoskeletal system	67	14	21

Data from reference 7. Reproduced with permission of Lippincott/Harper and Row.

Table 12-2
Complications Associated with the Treatment of Major Pelvic Disruptions

Complications	No. of Patients	Died
Urinary tract infection*	30	1
Atelectasis	24	7
Chest/lung infection	18	9
Disseminated intravascular coagulopathy†	10	5
Thromboembolism	9	3
Adult respiratory disease syndrome†	8	3
Major vessel injury	3	1
Peripheral nerve injury	3	0
Septicemia	4	4
Others	7	—

*Nosocomial infection, especially urinary, is commonplace.
†Associated mortality of 50%.
Data from reference 7. Reproduced with permission of Lippincott/Harper & Row.

In the series of McMurtry et al, all patients were treated nonsurgically for the pelvic fracture. They found no correlation between a specific type of fracture and obstetrical outcome, although they noted patients with bilateral pubic rami fractures had the worst obstetric sequelae.

There is little data on pelvic fractures in pregnancy. Speer and Peltier[8] studied the obstetrical outcome of 62 cases of pelvic fracture occurring either before or during pregnancy (Table 12-3).

Diagnosis of pelvic trauma in pregnancy can in some cases be difficult. Complaints of pelvic pain are common in pregnancy. The effects of "relaxin" on pelvic ligament structures is well known.[9]

Nontraumatic diastasis of the pubic symphysis associated with local tenderness is common in pregnancy. The average width of the symphysis pubis is 4 mm in nonpregnant women and 8 mm in pregnant women. Traumatic separation of the

Table 12-3
Summary of the Obstetrical Outcome of 11 Cases Reported Plus That of 51 Additional Cases Extracted from Published Reports

Patients (No.)	Live Births (No.)		Fetal Loss (No.)
	Vaginal	*Caesarean*	
Pregnant at time of fracture: 51.5% (32)	50% (16)	15.5% (5)	34.5% (11)
Fracture prior to pregnancy: 48.5% (30)	53.5% (16)	36.5% (11)	10% (3)
100% (62)	51.5% (32)	26% (16)	22.5% (14)

Data are from reference 8. Reproduced with permission of Williams & Wilkins.

pubic symphysis has been reported with trauma "as mild as running" in late pregnancy.[10]

Treatment of minor diastasis of the pubic symphysis is primarily rest and a pelvic binder for support. Traction with a pelvic sling may occasionally be necessary in more symptomatic cases.

Pubic symphysis separations greater than 40 mm are often associated with significant pelvic trauma and may require reduction with external fixation. Posttraumatic fusion of the symphysis will preclude future vaginal delivery.

Adequate radiographic assessment is essential in the treatment of pelvic fractures. Pennal and Sutherland[11] described a radiographic technique consisting of three anterior-posterior projections with the patient in the supine position: 1) a true anterior-posterior position, 2) an inlet projection with the x-ray beam directed 30° off vertical from the head, and 3) outlet projecting with the x-ray beam directed 30° off vertical from the feet (Figure 12-3).

Computerized tomography scanning gives a significant amount of information especially for acetabular fractures with relatively low collimated radiation.[11] Recent technological im-

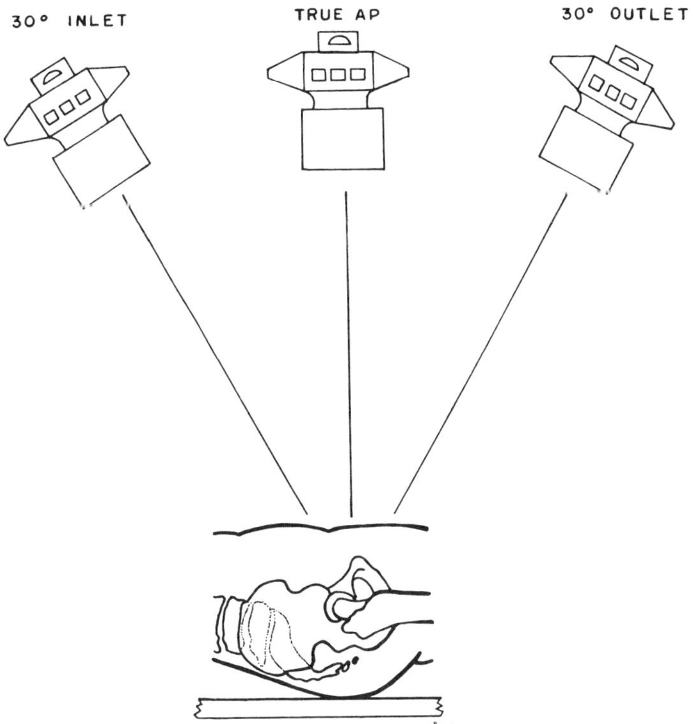

Figure 12-3 Technique for series of three radiological views of the pelvis. (Adapted from Mears DC: *External Skeletal Fixation.* Baltimore, Williams & Wilkins, with permission.)

provements have decreased radiation exposure to significantly less than regular tomography. The radiation is limited and collimated to the areas studied.

Acetabular fractures require 45° of internal and external oblique roentgenograms to evaluate the anterior and posterior columns of the acetabulum.

Treatment

Most pelvic fractures are stable and as such require only symptomatic treatment: bed rest until comfortable, analgesics and progressive ambulation to tolerance with crutches.

The x-rays in Figure 12-4 are those of a 19-year-old woman who was four months pregnant when struck by an automobile and sustained a minimally displaced pubic ramus fracture. After three weeks of bed rest, she was discharged comfortably ambulating with crutches.

Unstable pelvic fractures are often associated with significant residual trauma as well as significant pelvic bleeding.

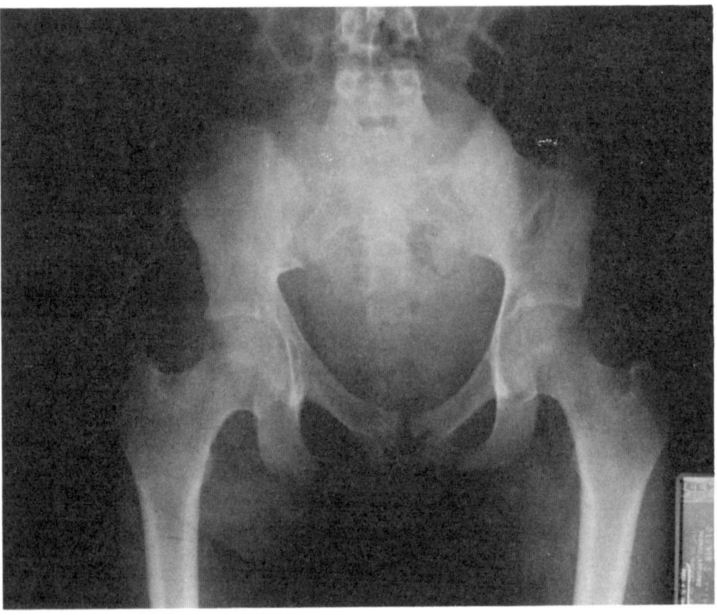

Figure 12-4 X-rays of 19-year-old woman, four months pregnant, with pubic ramus fracture after a motor vehicle accident.

Mears[12] has shown a significant decrease in blood loss associated with pelvic fractures when treated with external skeletal fixation.

External skeletal fixation decreases fracture pain, allows mobilization so vital for pulmonary function, and will prevent further damage from sharp bone fragments.

The Pittsburgh triangular frame (Figure 12-5) uses two clusters of 5-mm blunt external fixation pins placed by the open technique into the anterior iliac crest. These are held together by a series of ball joints and connecting rods.[12]

THE HIP

Hip dislocation requires a significant force and is usually associated with motor vehicle or industrial accidents. A fall

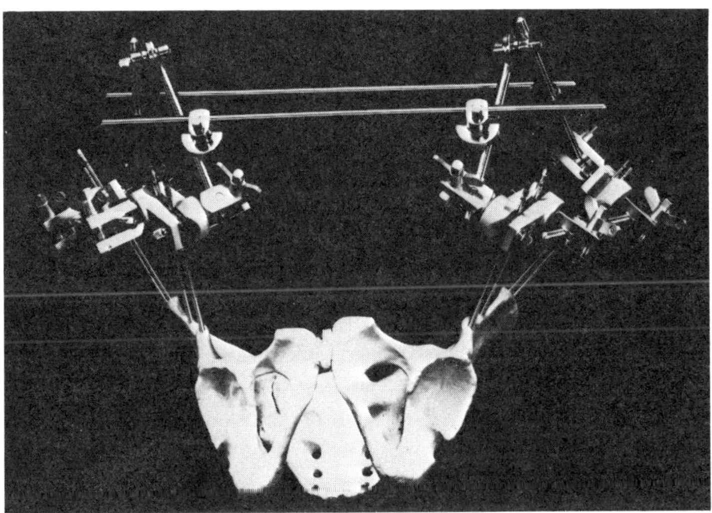

Figure 12-5 The Pittsburgh pelvic frame used in the management of many unstable pelvic fractures. (Courtesy Howmedica, Inc., Rutherford, NJ.)

from a height also produces this injury. A direct blow to the flexed knee with the hip flexed is a common mechanism of injury. Trauma of the knee or femur should alert the physician to carefully examine the hip. Closed reduction should be done as soon as possible with adequate anesthesia. The longer the delay in reduction, the greater the incidence of aseptic necrosis of the femoral head. The blood supply to the femoral head is via the capsular vessels which are compromised in the hip dislocation. Pregnancy alone has also been associated with aseptic necrosis.[13] Most simple hip dislocations are stable after reduction. Post reduction care should include three weeks of bed rest followed by partial weight bearing on crutches for nine weeks. Computerized tomography scanning of fracture dislocation of the hip can very accurately outline the congruity of reduction and evaluate the possibility of interarticular bone fragments, which may or may not be visible on regular radiographs. Interarticular bone fragments should be expediously surgically removed. Posterior acetabular fracture fragments should be reduced to prevent instability. Surgical approaches requiring a prone position should be avoided if possible because of pressure to the uterus and its compression of the inferior vena cava.

FRACTURES OF THE HIP AND FEMUR

Subcapital and transcervical fractures are rare in young adults. These are associated with high velocity injuries to the immediate area. They are also associated with an increased incidence of aseptic necrosis of the femoral head, a condition also associated with pregnancy.[13] As such open reduction and internal fixation should be done as soon as possible regardless of the trimester of pregnancy. X-ray shielding of the fetus should be attempted during evaluation and surgical treatment.

Intertrochanteric fractures and subintertrochanteric fractures should be fixed surgically, although in the last several weeks of pregnancy, skeletal traction while awaiting delivery may be indicated.

Fractures of the midshaft of the femur and below may be treated surgically or with skeletal traction and cast bracing. Maintenance of a supine position as required in skeletal traction for femoral fractures produces the problem of vena caval obstruction by the uterus in the second and especially the third trimester. With bed rest in late pregnancy, there is also an increased incidence of phlebitis, thrombal embolism, and pulmonary atelectasis secondary to a high uterus pressing on the diaphragm.

Physical therapy with cast bracing should emphasize transfer from bed to wheelchair and possibly to a walker. As gait stability is compromised in the second and third trimester, ambulation with crutches is not advisable in the pregnant patient immobilized with cast brace or long leg cast.

Hip spica casts can be modified to accommodate an expanding abdomen. They are not compatible with delivery. If they must be used during pregnancy a plan can be made for their removal and application of traction for labor and delivery.

The classical method of several weeks of skeletal traction before cast bracing or spica casting should be set aside in favor of early mobilization with surgical rigid fixation or early cast bracing popularized by Mooney et al.[14]

Early mobilization and bringing the patient into an upright position for pulmonary ventilation and pulmonary toilet is especially vital in the obese and/or multiply traumatized patient.

KNEE TRAUMA

With fractures of the femur or tibia, the knee requires close examination for associated trauma, commonly ligamentous rupture.

Weight increase and gait instability as well as the effects of relaxin all predispose the pregnant women to ligamentous injury. In the face of significant pain and swelling adequate evaluation of the knee may require anesthesia and arthroscopy. Pregnancy should not be a factor to deter surgical repair of ligamentous injury to the knee.

Postrepair immobilization in a cast brace with control of range of motion has been shown to give superior end results as compared with the standard method of postoperative immobilization with a long leg cast and no early controlled motion.

Physical activity and the patient expectation for sports activities are considered in the management of isolated ligamentous ruptures. Sedentary nonathletic patients with isolated anterior cruciate or medially collateral ligament ruptures can be managed nonoperatively with cast immobilization.

THE LEG

Most tibial fractures can be handled with closed reduction and cast immobilization. One must keep in mind that the increased peripheral venous pressure of late pregnancy predisposes to increased bleeding and compartment syndromes.

Surgical intervention in tibial shaft fractures in which satisfactory alignment cannot be maintained by closed casting techniques can be delayed two to three weeks if parturition is imminent.

Closed intramedullary fixation with tibial Ender's nails or "pins and plaster" fixation allow rapid mobilization of the patient with minimal surgery.

Cast bracing is especially advantageous for the pregnant patient in that it allows greater mobilization earlier than with other techniques.[14]

REFERENCES

1. Noland L, Cornwell HE: Fractures of the pelvis. *JAMA* 1930; 94:174.
2. Noland L, Cornwell HE: Acute fractures of the pelvis. *Surg Gynecol Obstet* 1923; 56:522.
3. Eliason E, Johnson JS: Fractures of the pelvis. *Clin Orthop North Am* 1937;17:1571.
4. Gustillo RV: *Management of Open Fractures and Their Complications*. Philadelphia, The WB Saunders Co, 1982.

5. Sutherland S: *Nerves and Nerve Injuries*. Baltimore, The Williams & Wilkins Co, 1968.
6. Tile M, Pennal G: Pelvic disruption: Principles of management. *Clin Orthop Rel Res* 1980;151:56.
7. McMurtry R, Walton D, Dickinson D, et al: Pelvic disruption in the polytraumatized patient: A management protocol. *Clin Orthop Rel Res* 1980;151:22.
8. Speer DP, Peltier LP: Pelvic fractures and pregnancy. *J Trauma* 1972;12:474.
9. Abramson D, Roberts S, Wilson P: Relaxation of the pelvic joints in pregnancy. *Surg Gynecol Obstet* 1934;58:595.
10. Splain SH, Edwards B: Traumatic separation of pubic symphysis with heterotropic bone. *Orthop Rev* 1982;11:111.
11. Pennal GF, Sutherland GO: Fractures of the pelvis (a motion picture). American Academy of Orthopaedic Surgery. Film Library, 1961.
12. Mears DC: *External Skeletal Fixation*. Baltimore, The Williams & Wilkins Co, 1983.
13. Epps C: *Complications of Orthopaedic Surgery*. Philadelphia, JB Lippincott, 1978.
14. Mooney V, Nichel V, Harvey JP et al: Cast brace treatment for fractures of the distal part of the femur. *J Bone Joint Surg* 1970; 52A:1563.

CHAPTER 13

NEUROLOGICAL INJURIES IN PREGNANCY

ROGER W. COUNTEE
JAMES P. THOMPSON
BUEL A. STAGGERS

Accidental and/or violent injuries represent the leading causes of death in Americans in the first four decades of life.[1] In spite of the fact that accurate statistics are painfully lacking, it is estimated that central nervous system trauma, ie, brain and/or spinal cord injury, is the primary cause of death or at least a major contributor to mortality in 60% to 75% of these fatal injuries.[1,2] Moreover, the true incidence of nonfatal central nervous system injuries or peripheral nerve injuries with or without permanent or nonpermanent neurologic sequelae is unknown. Although a heavy male preponderance is recognized to exist in the statistics for head injury, this does not appear to be the case for spinal cord injuries.[3] Furthermore, the major role of vehicular accidents in these statistics[1,4] and injuries incurred in the workplace[5] where women are becoming more ubiquitous have rendered the woman of child-bearing age increasingly more at risk for neurologic injuries. Consequently, neurologic injury during pregnancy is not at all rare.

Because of the complexity of the nervous system as well as its dominant position in determining both survival and quality of that survival in the trauma patient, it is understandable that most nonneurologic specialists feel a great sense of urgency, if not frank panic, when confronted with a patient with such injuries. Understandably, these trepidations are compounded when the trauma victim is pregnant and the potential for 200% failure is clearly recognized. Nevertheless, since the measures instituted by the first physician called upon to treat these injuries are often pivotal in determining their outcome, it is imperative that the nonneurologic specialist have a comfortable working knowledge of how to recognize and stabilize both the obvious and the occult neurologic injuries that one may encounter in the pregnant patient.

CRANIO-CEREBRAL INJURIES

Mechanisms of Injury and Definitions of Lesions

Important to one's ability to diagnose and manage head injuries is a working familiarity with the biomechanics that cause the various lesions as well as the correct terminology used to describe them. Fundamental is the recognition that indirect mechanical forces applied to the brain may be as devastating as direct blunt impact blows to the head with which we are most familiar. Since the cerebral hemispheres are to some extent suspended within the cranium in cerebrospinal fluid, relative movements of the brain within and independent of the skull may occur. This movement may result from a direct impact to the skull, from indirect forces such as rotational or torque forces transmitted to the brain by tangential blows to the face or cranium, or from sudden accelerations or decelerations of the head and/or trunk. In contrast, the brainstem, in which lies the reticular activating system, which sends constant volleys of electrical impulse up to arouse and maintain wakefulness of the cerebral cortex, is tethered to the base of the skull by the cranial nerves and the major arteries and veins that irrigate and drain the brain respectively. Consequently, both direct and indirect forces that cause mass movement of the brain within the skull or the skull around the brain will most often have a shearing or torque effect upon the brainstem and/or its blood supply.

It is this torsion or stretching of the brainstem which impairs the electrical physiology of the reticular activating system and the consequent impairment of an individual's alertness or wakefulness. This phenomenon is common and may vary in degrees of severity. Transient electrical dysfunction of the brainstem's reticular acting system not associated with morphologic changes in the brain results in the classical clinical picture of the concussion. A cerebral concussion is defined as a clinical syndrome that results from mechanical forces and is characterized by a transient impairment of neural function, eg, alteration of alertness, disturbances in vision such as "seeing stars or flashing spots," disequilibrium, giddiness, etc. The impaired state of consciousness that results from a concussion is characteristically brief and usually lasts for only seconds or at most a few minutes. The relatively evanescent nature of a cerebral concussion can be appreciated when one thinks of the paresthesias and weakness experienced in the fingers and forearm after a blow to the "funny bone" and the ulnar nerve has been concussed at the elbow. Consequently, any patient who remains unconscious for more than 5 or 10 minutes or awakens after a brief period of unconsciousness to only later become lethargic or stuporous, or has a focal neurologic deficit, must by definition have more than just a concussion.

With the movement of the cerebral hemispheres themselves within the skull the brain may glide over the rock hard surface of the skull base and be bruised to varying extents. In these circumstances the tips of the temporal lobes may be impaled against the sharp edges of the petrous ridges or the undersurface of the frontal poles may be bruised as they slide over the roughened roofs of the orbits. Consequently, these regions of the brain are particularly disposed to injury regardless of whether the trauma is a direct blow to the head or due to indirect forces. The bruising of the brain is termed a contusion and is indeed a structural alteration of the superficial layers of the brain as opposed to the electrophysiologic phenomenon of concussion. A contusion is characterized by hemorrhage, necrosis, and edema of the brain's surface. Some degree of cerebral contusion invariably occurs below the site of a severe direct impact, whether or not there is an overlying skull fracture, and is termed a coup contusion. In contrast, however, when the moving head strikes a fixed or slower moving object, such as what happens during a fall or a collision, often the most severe or perhaps the only area of brain contusion may commonly be diametrically opposite to the site of skull impact and is termed a contracoup contusion.

Although a cerebral contusion may frequently accompany a cerebral concussion, it is the location and extent of the cerebral contusion that determine its clinical manifestations. That is to say, that only if this type of injury involves the primary motor, sensory, or visual cortex or the pyramidal tracts at the midbrain peduncles, etc, will it be associated with the more familiar focal neurologic deficits or hemiparesis, hemisensory loss, visual field cuts, etc. It must be remembered, however, that the poles of the frontal and temporal lobes, which are particularly predisposed to contusions as well as lacerations, are not the sites of these aforementioned functions. Memory and emotional coloring are some of the functions housed within the temporal lobes. Psychic motivation, volition, and social inhibition are some of the functions of the premotor frontal poles. It is the dysfunction of these structures that effects changes in personality and memory which are frequently seen in the head injured patient after she has recovered from her brief loss of consciousness from a concussion or from a prolonged stupor secondary to a more severe brain injury. In fact, the impairment of memory, or amnesia is frequently concomitant to, if not indeed a hallmark of, a concussion. Amnesia for events after the injury is termed retrograde. It is not at all uncommon that amnesia may be the only physical clue available to the clinician that his patient has sustained a concussion. In general the severity and length of the amnesia parallels the severity of the temporal lobe injury.

Almost invariably with severe head injuries of any type and particularly those that result in cerebral contusions, there is associated a degree of congestion or swelling of cerebral tissues. This brain swelling or cerebral edema is, likewise, a true morphologic change that is particularly prone to occur in cerebral white matter. Depending on its extent, the electrical transmission along the nerve axons which the white matter serves to insulate and, thereby, facilitate electrical transmissions may be impaired, and a consequent neurologic deficit may be clinically manifest despite anatomically intact neurons. The site of the edema, which may be focal, multifocal, or diffuse as well as its severity determines the clinical picture. Cerebral edema may not reach its maximum severity until 72 hours or more after the injury and thus may be a cause for delayed neurologic deterioration. On the other hand it may rapidly fulminate in less than 30 minutes, in which case the outcome is usually fatal. Cerebral edema may be tremendously aggravated by hypoxia, hypercarbia, hyperpyrexia, systemic hypotension or hypertension, sepsis, impaired cerebral venous drainage, etc. Fulminant cerebral edema is a frequent cause of profound neurlogic deficits and may cause shifting of portions of the brain within the various cranial compartments, secondary compression of vital brainstem centers, and consequent impairment of central cardiovascular and respiratory centers and death. The clinical picture of cerebral edema is often indistinguishable from that caused by a traumatic intracranial hematoma with which it may frequently be associated.

Intracranial hemorrhages may occur within the brain parenchyma itself, over the brain's surface below the dura, or above the dura below a fracture site in the skull. *Intraparenchymal* or *intracerebral hemorrhages* are often the consequence of what begins as extensive cerebral contusions and, therefore, tend to occur either beneath the site of an impact or in the predisposed areas of the brain previously described. *Acute traumatic subdural* hematomas are usually caused by tearing of the blood vessels on the surface of the brain or by frank lacerations of the brain substance. Both of these lesions are the consequence of tremendously violent injuries and usually appear as a profound neurologic deficit with marked impairment of consciousness promptly after the injury or shortly thereafter, within minutes to at most a few hours. Acute extradural hemorrhages most often occur below a fracture of the cranial vault and separate the dura from the skull. Although the clinician is particularly alert to this possibility when the skull fracture is seen to be near to or traversing a major vascular structure such as the middle meningeal artery or the major dural sinuses, it is important to note that the major bleeding in these situations most frequently comes from the fractured bone fragments themselves. Consequently, all large or significantly displaced skull fractures must be recognized as potential sites for an extradural hematoma. Since the brain parenchyma is not directly injured in many of these cases, manifest neurologic deficits most often result from extraaxial compression by the expanding clot. The briskness of the bleeding and the rapidity with which a sizeable hematoma develops, as well as the cerebral localization, determine the clinical picture. Consequently, a brief loss of consciousness or impairment of alertness initially after impact and then subsequent neurologic deterioration is frequently seen in the clinical evaluation of these lesions.

Skull fractures derive their importance from essentially two major reasons. 1) Their presence alone documents that a severe violent energy has been imparted to the head, and the size and degree of the displacement of fracture fragments (comminution) tend to parallel the magnitude of the applied mechanical forces. 2) The location of the fracture gives clues as to the various structures that possibly may also be injured: a) important regions of the cerebral cortex such as speech centers, motor and sensory areas, visual cortex, etc; b) various vascular structures including those at the skull base such as the carotid arteries and the cavernous sinus, the jugular foramen and its contents, etc; c) the paranasal sinuses and their potential as possible sources of cerebrospinal fluid leakage and contamination and the subsequent evolution of meningitis; d) the cranial nerves at the base of the skull, etc. Skull fractures that lie below an overlying scalp laceration or avulsion (compound fractures) are also recognized for their potential for the subsequent development of intracranial suppuration. It is important to note that in the course of fracturing the skull much of the violent energy of an impact is absorbed in the process. Consequently, fracturing the skull tends to exert a protective effect for the brain to some extent. However, the corollary to this is that the worst parenchymal brain injuries frequently occur in the absence of a skull fracture. Therefore, the physician should not be lulled into a false sense of security by reportedly negative skull x-rays, particularly when the history of the severity of the injury and/or the clinical signs indeed suggest a significant brain injury.

Intracranial pressure is routinely elevated when the volume of the intracranial contents is increased. Consequently, intracranial hypertension occurs not only in cases of intracranial hematomas, but whenever brain swelling occurs alone or with an associated intracranial clot. It is recognized that differential pressure gradients within the various intracranial compartments are the cause of segments of brain to shift or herniate across the midline, into the incisura of the tentorium cerebelli, or downward through the foramen magnum and cause compression of the brainstem. However, in the circumstance of an acute and generalized or global increase in intracranial pressure in which the pressure does not approximate systemic diastolic blood pressure and herniation has not occurred and is not imminent, the consequences of intracranial hypertension are not clear, and the merits of its treatment are controversial.

Evaluation and Management of the Head Injured Pregnant Woman

Although a basic understanding of the biomechanics and patterns of craniocerebral injury is fundamental, the history of the traumatic event and the neurologic examination of the patient are equally as important in recognizing the presence and manifestations of the variety of lesions that are possible—obvious or occult. A baseline neurologic status, which should be documented by the first physician or paramedic who attends the injured patient, is crucial in making serial objective determinations of whether the patient is deteriorating or improving spontaneously or as a result of therapy. Crucial is the determination of the patient's initial level of wakefulness. In this regard it is much better to describe what the patient does, eg, "sleeps when unattended, but easily rouses upon command to converse appropriately with dysarthric sentence fragments and moves all four limbs briskly, left more than right" as opposed to simply using poorly defined adjectives alone such as stuporous, comatose, semiconscious, etc.

In addition, language function, vision, and the content of the wakefulness should be noted and can be ascertained in the course of taking the history from the patient about the circumstances surrounding the traumatic event as well as in the course of an oral review of organ systems. Brainstem function is assessed by determining the level of alertness and also by testing cranial nerve function particularly the size, symmetry, and reactivity of the pupils, as well as voluntary and/or elicited eye movements, etc. Voluntary, involuntary, or absent movements in the limbs and loss of sensation in the face and limbs should be looked for and described. Muscle tone and the ease with which deep tendon reflexes are elicited and their symmetry should also be recorded. The presence or absence of abnormal reflexes such as an extensor plantar response (Babinski sign) should also be specifically noted. Equally important is the determination of the vital signs including blood pressure, pulse, temperature, and respiratory rate and rhythm. Frequently, these parameters will give clues as to the presence, location, and course of a neurologic injury or perhaps suggest that the neurological picture may be consequent to or compounded by an extracranial systemic disorder.

In an attempt to reduce the confusion that often arises from an ambiguous description of a patient's level of consciousness, the so-called Glascow coma scale (Table 13-1) was introduced in 1974 in an effort to standardize these descriptions.[6] It is not and, moreover it does not purport to be a description of neurologic

Table 13-1
The Glascow Coma Scale*

Category	Observed Response	Score†
Eye opening	Spontaneous	4
	To speech	3
	To pain	2
	None	1
Best verbal response	Oriented	5
	Confused	4
	Inappropriate	3
	Incomprehensible	2
	None	1
Best motor response	Obeying	6
	Localizing	5
	Normal flexion	4
	Abnormal flexion	3
	Extending	2
	None	1

*After Teasdale and Jennet.[6]
†The total score is an aggregate of the number in each of the three categories. The maximum is 15; the minimum is 3.

status and is meant only to describe a patient's level of wakefulness by scoring three simple functions: 1) eye opening, 2) motor response, and 3) the ability to speak. Although this scale may have great usefulness for the nonneurologic specialist, in these authors opinion it cannot be used to replace a well written and detailed description of a patient's level of consciousness and her neurologic status.

Minor Head Injuries

Superficial injuries to the face and scalp are common injuries, which most often are not accompanied by significant cranial or cerebral trauma. If there is no history of severe impact, skull penetration, or loss of consciousness and a normal neurologic examination then the physician can usually be comfortable with simply managing the lacerations and/or avulsions of the scalp according to standard surgical principles of vigorous debridement and thorough irrigation of the wound followed by meticulous reapproximation of the wound edges. In such situations the hair should be shaved about 5 cm from the wound edges to facilitate wound toilet and repair as well as the application of a suitable dressing. It must be remembered that because of the luxuriant blood supply to the scalp, bleeding from a relatively small scalp laceration can result in surprisingly profuse bleeding and substantial blood loss, which may alone be cause for hypovolemic hypotension and an indication for transfusion. Scalp bleeding can initially be controlled with firm digital pressure to the wound edges or compressive dressings until the definitive repair. However, wound repair for reapproximation as well as for hemostasis should be done expeditiously as soon as the clinical situation permits and should not be deferred until the arrival of the neurosurgeon or after skull x-rays are taken. Since the ability to diagnose the presence or absence of a skull fracture by blind palpation through a laceration with a finger or probe is notoriously inaccurate, we condemn this practice since it may introduce contamination into a wound where none previously existed. Plain skull x-rays are not an imperative in these situations, and these patients may be sent home with reliable family observers who have been informed about the important signs and symptoms of worsening neurologic function (Figure 13-1).

Moderately Severe Head Injuries

This category of injury would include linear skull fractures, minor fractures of the face and/or orbits, and a brief loss of consciousness (concussion) without manifest neurologic deficit other than posttraumatic amnesia. In these situations the history of the type of injury, the force of the impact, or the loss of consciousness merits obtaining skull x-rays and possibly roentgenograms of the facial bones and orbits after scalp lacerations

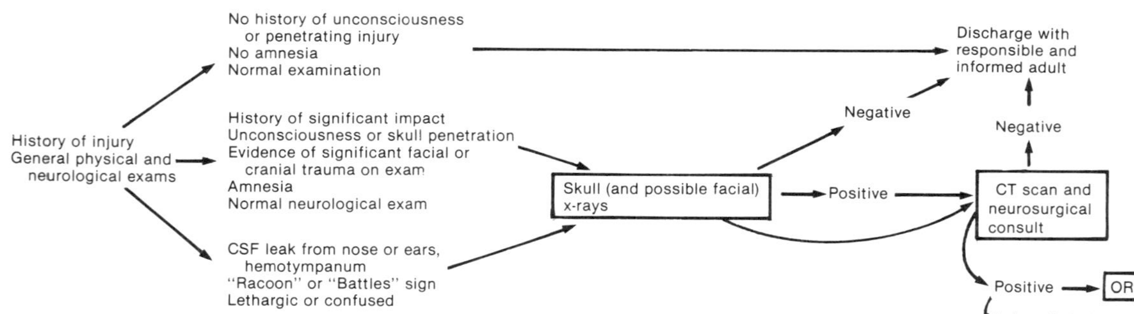

Figure 13-1 Acute head injury management in the pregnant female: the conscious patient. Neurological consultation should be obtained at any point where the emergency treating physician is unsure, although the results of skull x-rays and CT scan are most helpful to the neurosurgical opinion.

have been repaired. Neurosurgical consultation is appropriate to determine whether computerized tomography (CT) scan is indicated and whether operative intervention is necesssary. Uncomplicated cerebral concussion and/or linear nondisplaced skull fractures require no treatment, but their occurrence indicates a significant head injury and demands observation of the patient for at least 24 hours by either reliable and informed family or medical personnel and sequential outpatient follow-up.

Severe Head Injuries

Major facial fractures, penetrating injuries, depressed skull fractures, leakage of cerebrospinal fluid from the nose or ears, hemotympanum, sustained impairment of alertness, prominent changes in personality or memory, and other manifest neurologic deficits together or independently suggest a high possibility of a severe intracranial injury and the probable need for neurosurgical intervention. If no other injuries are present, then roentgenograms of the skull and facial bones as well as a plain scan should be done expeditiously after the baseline neurologic examination is documented and the patient's condition is stabilized. The location and degree of displacement of fracture fragments determine the need for neurosurgical intervention in the operating theater or in the emergency room. The CT scan will document the presence of an associated intracranial mass lesion and will discriminate between edema, contusion, and intracranial hematomas. Although the neurosurgeon must determine the necessity of operation, the timing of such a procedure as well as the role of adjunctive therapy must be jointly decided upon by the neurosurgeon and the obstetrician.

Extremely Severe Head Injuries

This category of patients includes those in which there is a marked impairment of wakefulness or progressing stupor, a prominent neurologic deficit, pupillary enlargement and/or asymmetry, abnormal attitudes or posturing of the limbs, large open wounds of the cranium, etc. The vital signs may also frequently be abnormal with a slow pulse, abnormally slow or rapid or arrhythmic respirations, and a rising blood pressure. If there are associated injuries to the thoracic and/or the abdominal viscera, including the gravid uterus, or major fractures, there is usually tachycardia and hypotension. In any event, the arrival of such a patient should promptly activate a well-ordered and standardized series of therapeutic and diagnostic events (Figure 13-2).

The first priority of management is the establishment and maintenance of an adequate and secure airway by prompt endotracheal intubation in which extension of the neck is carefully avoided. Hyperventilation and hyperoxygenation are induced in an effort to keep the pCO_2 between 24 and 28 torr and the pO_2 in excess of 85 torr, and initial arterial blood gas samples are obtained. Simultaneously, adqeuate arterial perfusion is established by infusion of intravenous fluids and/or blood as indicated, and obvious and accessible sites of hemorrhage are promptly controlled. The head and neck are immobilized as a unit until portable x-rays have excluded an associated cervical spine injury, which occurs in approximately 6% of these patients.[2] A rapid examination to establish a baseline neurologic status and to determine other sites of injury is made, and treatment of immediately life-threatening conditions such as pneumothorax or hemothorax are promptly initiated. The abdominal viscera are examined, and the status of the gravid uterus and fetus is assessed. Obvious extremity fractures are immobilized, and a urinary catheter is inserted.

Portable x-rays of the skull and cervical spine as well as the chest and abdomen and sites of suspected fractures should then be performed. Once spinal fractures have been excluded it is helpful to lay the pregnant patient on her side to reduce the effect of the gravid uterus on retarding venous return from the legs. In addition, the patient's head should be elevated 30° to 45° in an effort to facilitate venous drainage of the brain and

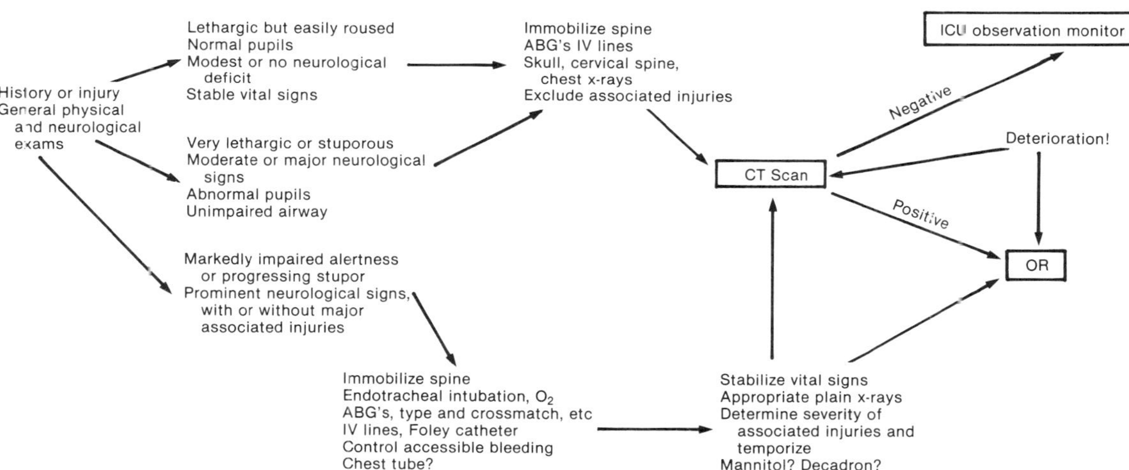

Figure 13-2 Acute head injury management in the pregnant female: the neurologically impaired and/or unconscious patient. The neurosurgeon is consulted upon patient's arrival to ER. However, physical assessment as well as temporizing and diagnostic measures are initiated promptly.

thereby improve intracranial vascular congestion and reduce increased intracranial pressure.

In the patient with a profound impairment of consciousness and/or a rapidly deteriorating neurologic status, mannitol (0.5 to 1.0 g/kg), should be rapidly infused over 15 to 30 minutes. Urinary output should be closely monitored, and 1000 to 2000 mL of urine in 30 to 45 minutes after infusion is expected when a good pharmacologic response to this osmotic diuretic has occurred. Balanced salt solutions, usually 5% dextrose in 0.45% normal saline or lactated Ringer's solution, should be given judiciously as the clinical picture dictates. If no major source of volume loss exists, then it is advisable to restrict total fluid intake to 1800 to 2000 mL/24 hours. Steroids, usually dexamethasone (20 mg to as much as 100 mg), are given as an intravenous bolus. Antibiotics for open head wounds or basal skull fractures with obvious leakage of cerebrospinal fluid are not routinely given and are reserved for only those wounds where gross contamination is evident. Narcotics or sedatives are never given because they may not only further impair alertness, but may also cause pupillary changes and respiratory depression. Although a seizure may accompany or follow upon the heels of an impact head injury, anticonvulsant drugs are rarely indicated in the emergency room situation.

Only after the vital functions have been stabilized is consideration given to moving the injured patient out of the emergency room and into the CT scan suite or to the operating theater. Although major thoracic and/or abdominal injuries, including a ruptured uterus, may take medical priority over a brain injury, it is clearly preferred to obtain a CT scan if at all possible to establish the site, nature, and extent of the cerebral lesion. A more informed neurosurgical judgment can then be made as to the necessity and timing of a cranial operation as well as nonsurgical treatment alternatives. The proper assignment of therapeutic priorities can best be accomplished by mutual agreement between the obstetrician and the neurosurgeon as well as the other surgical specialists involved.

NEUROLOGICAL PROGNOSIS AFTER HEAD INJURY AND OBSTETRIC COMPLICATIONS

Although the fate of the severely head injured patient and that of her unborn fetus may indeed be sealed at the moment of the initial injury, it is now recognized that this is true in far fewer patients than was heretofore believed. Experience has shown that if a patient has talked at any time after the initial injury then totally irrecoverable brain injury from the impact cannot be assumed. The majority of patients who have talked and then died have been demonstrated at autopsy to have had avoidable or treatable factors that contributed to or caused their demise. It is believed that a similar situation has existed in many of the patients who have not talked as well. The most common avoidable or treatable neurologic factors are delayed recognition and removal of an intracranial hematoma and/or the ineffective management of brain swelling. The most common extracranial factors are hypoxia and systemic hypotension, common concomitants in the multiply injured patient and particularly true in victims of vehicular accidents. In addition, it has long been recognized that youthful age and previous good health are extremely important factors that influence a favorable outcome. Consequently, there is no question that the head-injured pregnant woman demands an astute, energetic, aggressive, and optimistic therapeutic posture.

It is an accepted clinical maxim that under no circumstances should the life of the mother be jeopardized by the fact that she is pregnant. Consequently, one should not hesitate to perform necessary x-rays, CT scans, general anesthesia, and cranial surgery. This should not be misconstrued to mean, however, that the judicious selection of x-rays and well-reasoned treatment decisions can be replaced by indiscriminate disregard for the fetus. Fortunately, the same measures indicated for the treatment of a cerebral injury, via, a perfect airway, prevention of hypoxia and hypotension, moderate hypocarbia, etc are likewise indicated for fetal well-being. Although formerly recommended by many neurosurgeons, severe dehydration, hypovolemia, and hypothermia are no longer considered appropriate. Since mannitol's dehydrating effect on the amniotic fluid is similar to its effect on the brain, maternal plasma osmolarity should not be allowed to exceed 10% more than normal, and the repeated use of this diuretic should be avoided. Although high-dose corticosteroids have frequently been used throughout pregnancies without obvious ill effects upon the fetus, the exact effect of high dose dexamethasone upon the fetus is unknown. However, it is believed to have a positive effect on fetal lung maturation.

When multiple seizures follow a severe head injury or when a preinjury seizure disorder exists, anticonvulsant therapy is an imperative. Pregnancy alone may often initiate seizures and/or make seizure control difficult. However, this can be circumvented by intravenous administration of the anticonvulsant medication and monitoring of drug plasma levels. All of the anticonvulsant drugs, save for carbamazepine, have been reported to have some teratogenic effects, and many have been suggested to be a cause of increased perinatal mortality and an increased incidence of abnormal fetal and maternal bleeding with delivery.[7–9] The control of seizures is a paramount objective in these situations, however, and phenytoin continues to be a first-line drug in pregnancy. Monitoring of maternal and fetal clotting parameters and preparations for the possibility of a complicated delivery should, therefore, be automatic in these situations.

When the unfortunate circumstance of an irrecoverable brain injury and cerebral death occurs in the pregnant head injury victim a potentially viable fetus may become the medical priority. With life support systems, optimal nutrition, and attentive medical care the mother and her pregnancy can often be to sustained until delivery is deemed safe for the fetus. Although maternal hypothalamic and/or pituitary dysfunction may accompany such catastrophic brain injuries, with replacement therapy of cortisone, thyroid hormone, and vasopressin if needed, the pregnancy, good fetal growth, and a spontaneous vaginal delivery may proceed independent of the maternal pituitary.[10] Fetal head growth can be assessed with serial ultrasound examinations, and placental and maternal hormones can be monitored.[8] Delivery can be accomplished per vaginum after spontaneous or induced labor, or caesarean section may be elected. Although small birth weight and mild fetal distress may occur, the chances for the infant's good recovery and normal development appear to be excellent, and perhaps the dimensions of a potentially twofold tragedy can thereby be reduced.

The medicolegal considerations of defining and timing the mother's death as well as the legal ramifications of her death, particularly regarding inheritance, are superbly discussed in a recent review.[11]

SPINAL INJURY IN THE PREGNANT PATIENT

Emergency Evaluation and Management

Spinal injuries in the pregnant patient are most frequently the result of major falls or vehicular accidents and rarely secondary to penetrating injuries. Consequently, associated injuries are common and should be specifically looked for in these patients. The arrival of such patients to the emergency room should activate a systematic sequence of events to minimize the extent of the neural damage as well as the physiologic consequences of spinal cord dysfunction to other organ systems. Such patients should be immediately immobilized flat in the supine position, and suspected cervical spine fractures should be splinted with sand bags to both sides of the head and neck. Establishing and maintaining an airway with adequate ventilation is the number one priority, and careful nasotracheal intubation without moving the patient's head should be done promptly if the patient's ventilatory status is inadequate or at all suspect. Patients with lesions at or above C4 vertebral segments may have all respiratory muscles denervated and will usually not survive long enough to reach a hospital. Cervical cord injuries below C4 will usually spare the phrenic nerve outflow and allow diaphragmatic respirations in spite of the fact that thoracic musculature is paralyzed. However, in the presence of an enlarged gravid uterus diaphragmatic excursions are already compromised and are usually even further attenuated by the supine position. Consequently, ventilatory support is usually necessary in these situations and respiration parameters consistent with the stage of the pregnancy should be achieved. Although tracheostomy in the emergency room is rarely necessary, it may become indicated later as the clinical picture evolves.

Cervical cord injuries, the most frequent site of spinal injuries, not only result in paralysis and sensory loss in the trunk and limbs, but also interrupt sympathetic innervation (T1–L2) to thoracic, abdominal, and pelvic viscera. Loss of sympathetic tone to the heart and blood vessels results in bradycardia, diminished cardiac output, decreased peripheral arteriolar resistance, diminished venous tone, and consequent systemic hypotension. This situation is compounded further when the patient is in or beyond the 28th week of pregnancy and is placed in the supine position because the weight of the gravid uterus may impair venous return through the inferior vena cava and pelvic veins as well as impair arterial flow through the abdominal aorta. Consequently, the restoration and maintenance of an adequate circulation both arterial perfusion as well as venous return is the second medical priority in these patients. Although some authors have advocated the use of sympathomimetic drugs in these situations of postsympathectomy hypotension, experience has shown that these drugs may predispose patients to the development of acute pulmonary edema. Consequently, we recommend that every pregnant patient with a spinal cord injury have a Swan-Ganz catheter inserted, cardiac index parameters determined, and their circulatory status resuscitated with intravenous fluids either dextrose in 0.45% saline or lactated Ringer's solution. Elevation of the patient's legs, if the situation permits, may be helpful. However, the Trendelenberg position is contraindicated.

The evaluation of thoracic and abdominal viscera, including the uterus and its contents, and identifying additional fractures is then done expeditiously. A nasogastric tube and an indwelling urinary catheter should be inserted. As in the case of the head injured patient, life-threatening injuries to other organs may take priority over the neurologic injury. However, every effort should be made to perform a baseline neurologic evaluation as soon as possible. Portable x-rays should be done, without moving the patient if possible, and cross-table lateral films of the entire spinal column should be obtained as the patient's vital functions are being stabilized. It should be remembered that cervical spinal injuries frequently accompany head injuries, and thoracolumbar or lumbar fractures and/or dislocations are commonly associated with major injuries to thoracic and/or abdominal viscera as well as pelvic fractures. It is not uncommon, then, that major visceral injuries dominate the clinical picture in these emergency situations, and the detection of a spinal injury may be delayed unless the clinician has a heightened index of suspicion when confronted with these situations.

Definitive neurologic diagnosis usually requires the neurosurgeon who is consulted promptly in these cases. The need for additional x-ray views and/or other diagnostic tests is determined by the neurosurgeon and performed under his supervision. Ideally, any spinal cord compression by malaligned vertebral segments, acutely ruptured discs, or bony fracture fragments should be promptly relieved. Most often this can be done by skeletal traction with skull tongs in the more common situations of cervical fractures and/or dislocations. However, the less common situation of thoracic, thoracolumbar, or lumbar fractures and/or dislocations may often require operative reduction and internal fixation. After a definitive assessment treatment must be decided upon by the neurosurgeon and/or the orthopedic surgeon and the hierarchy of medical priorities can be appropriately established after discussion between them, the obstetrician, and the other involved surgical consultants.

Surgical Considerations and Obstetric Implications

If the fetus of the mother with acute spinal injury has not been injured by the trauma, then all of the nonoperative measures outlined for treating the mother are likewise beneficial for the child. If the fetus is sufficiently mature for delivery and thoracic or lumbar surgery is urgently needed, then caesarean section before such surgery should be considered. In contrast, operative reduction and fixation of cervical fractures and/or dislocations is not complicated by the protuberant uterus and can be easily performed while allowing the pregnancy to proceed without interruption. On the other hand, when the fetus is salvageable, but gestationally immature, the severity of the mother's neurologic deficit may influence therapeutic decisions. For example, if the mother is profoundly tetraplegic or paraplegic despite successful nonoperative reduction of an unstable fracture and/or dislocation and prolonged confinement to bed is anticipated because of the neurologic deficit, then satisfactory maintenance of spinal alignment may often be achieved with bed rest alone. This is best accomplished with the Roto-Rest bed, which effectively immobilizes patients in the supine position and therefore easily accommodates the gravid uterus. Because of its continous oscillations from side to side, however, it appears to effectively reduce the cardiopulmonary and other complications of prolonged bed rest and the supine position. The fetus can thus be allowed to mature to term. Delivery in the lithotomy position in these situations is contraindicated because it places the spine in kyphus and threatens cord compression. Although the Sims position is often advocated in these circumstances and is theoretically acceptable, it frequently is impractical. Consequently, elective caesarean section is most often the safer procedure in these circumstances.

In situations where the neurologic deficit from cord injury is modest or nil yet is threatened by an unstable fracture, then expeditious operative fixation is preferred to facilitate early mobilization of the patient and to begin rehabilitative measures promptly. In these cases the risks to the fetus of general anesthesia and major spinal surgery must be accepted in the best interest of the mother. Procedures on the cervical spine may be successfully done in the supine or sitting position. Operative approaches to the thoracic or lumbar spine can be done in the lateral position. If a body spica is necessary, an abdominal window must be fashioned, and the cast must be changed frequently to accommodate the growing fetus. Fortunately, a variety of external fixation devices are now available which may preclude the need for a body cast. In cases of stable or stabilized fractures or internally fixed fractures vaginal delivery is allowed.

Although the exact role of the spinal cord innervation to the female reproductive system is unclear, it is well documented that in spite of chronic denervation secondary to lesions in either peripheral nerves, the cauda equina, or the spinal cord itself, normal labor with effective uterine expulsion of the fetus per vaginum can indeed occur. The conscious sensation of pain in the uterus and adnexa is carried via afferent fibers travelling with the sympathetic nerves (hypogastric nerves) to and from T10 to L1 spinal cord segments. Consequently, cord injuries at or above these segments not only will result in motor and sensory loss to the distal trunk and limbs but also will result in painless labor that may go unrecognized as such by the patient and her obstetrician. In contrast, the conscious sensation of pain in the perineum, introitus, vaginal vault, and anus are carried via somatic afferent fibers in the pudendal nerve back to cord segments S2 to S5 (the conus medullaris situated at T12 to L1 vertebral bodies). The conscious sensation of fullness in the bladder and rectum travels with parasympathetic fibers via the pelvic nerve or Nervus erigens back to the conus as well (S3 to S5 cord segments). Efferent parasympathic fibers from these sacral segments of the conus are predominant in the propulsive contractions of the bladder and rectum. Somatic efferent fibers from the conus travel via the pudendal nerve (S3 to S5) and carry voluntary control to the external anal and vesicle sphincters as well as to the striated musculature of the pelvic floor.

Consequently, traumatic lesions of spinal elements below L1 will result in perineal anesthesia, which affords a painless episiotomy as well as relaxation of the pelvic floor and incontinence of urine and feces. However, the pain and the course of uterine contractions will be unaffected.

Although the spinal cord-injured pregnant woman may be beset with many problems, eg, chronic urinary tract infections, anemia, decubitii, leg and perineal muscle spasms, autonomic hyperreflexia (may mimic eclampsia), cardiac arrhythmias, labor before 40 weeks, a higher risk of fetal anomalies, stillbirths, or abortion, etc, in general a good pregnancy outcome may be expected if these complications are anticipated and properly managed.[12-14] Vaginal delivery is preferred unless there is an obstetric contraindication. Since catgut sutures are poorly absorbed by tetraplegics and paraplegics and buried sutures often cause sterile abscesses, episiotomies in these circumstances should be repaired with nonabsorbable sutures (silk, nylon, or steel). Subsequent pregnancies may be achieved with sexual counseling and without a higher risk of fetal difficulties, and capable and gratifying parenting may be enjoyed by the properly motivated mother with spinal injury.[12-15]

NERVE ROOT AND PERIPHERAL NERVE INJURIES IN PREGNANCY

Traumatic injuries to the cervical or lumbosacral roots may occur during pregnancy secondary to violent head or neck movements, collisions, or falls. Moreover, the hormonal, postural, and mechanical stresses of pregnancy are known to predispose to the herniation of lumbar discs during the pregnancy. Immobilization, bed rest, local heat and massage, and minor analgesics, if truly necessary, most often are effective in these situations, and myelography and spinal surgery can usually be deferred until the puerperium or later. Diazepam, a sedative and muscle relaxant commonly used in these situations, is contraindicated in pregnancy and during lactation.[16] If a neurologic deficit is profound – eg, loss of bowel and bladder control, a foot drop – or is progressively worsening, then spinal surgery should not be delayed but should be performed promptly in spite of the pregnancy.

It is well known that compression of peripheral nerves, nerve trunks, and/or the lumbosacral plexus may occur during labor and delivery. These injuries may be caused by the fetal head, the application of forceps, improper positioning in leg holders, or trauma and hematoma incurred during caesarean section. In addition, pregnancy is known to predispose to the development of certain entrapment neuropathies, eg, carpal tunnel syndrome with median nerve compression at the wrist, meralgia paresthetica secondary to compression of the lateral femoral cutaneous nerve by the inguinal ligament, etc. Fortunately, these conditions usually spontaneously remit after delivery; only uncommonly is operative correction indicated and certainly not during the pregnancy. Detailed reviews of the diagnosis and management of these disorders are available for the interested reader.[12,14,17]

In open injuries of peripheral nerves, emergency surgical repair is rarely an imperative, and certainly not when the wound is not closed primarily or is contaminated. However, when clean wounds are repaired initially, then primary repair of a visibly transected nerve is preferred if an optimal operating room situation exists. If circumstances are not optimal because of the clinical situation, eg, profuse hemorrhage from or occlusion of a major artery, if more life-threatening medical or surgical emergencies coexist, or if experienced personnel and equipment are not readily available, then primary nerve suture should be deferred. In this situation the status of the nerve should be determined, its proximal and distal ends should be marked with radiopaque wires or silver clips, and the ends should be held close together so that a large gap will not develop. Nerve repair is, therefore, delayed until a more optimal time and circumstances exist. When the anatomical status of the nerve is not known as with gunshot wounds, puncture or incisional wounds, or closed extremity fractures, serial neurologic examinations and electromyograms are helpful in determining the optimal therapy and the most appropriate timing of surgery, if any.

REFERENCES

1. Trunkey DD: Trauma. *Sci Am* 1983;249:28.
2. Gurdjian ES, Gurdjian ES: Acute head injuries. *Surg Gynecol Obstet* 1978;146:805.
3. Kalsbeek WD, McLaurin RL, Harris BSH III, et al: The national head and spinal cord injury survey: Major findings. *J Neurosurg* 1980;53:(suppl)S19.
4. Council on Scientific Affairs: Automobile related injuries: Components, trends, prevention. *JAMA* 1983;249:3216.
5. Division of Safety Research Report, NIOSH and CDC: Work related disorders. *JAMA* 1983;249:2301.
6. Teasdale G, Jennett B: Assessment of coma and impaired consciousness. A practical scale. *Lancet* 1974;2:81.
7. Philbert A, Dam M: The epileptic mother and her child. *Epilepsia* 1982;23:85.
8. Sampson MB, Peterson LP: Post traumatic coma during pregnancy. *Obstet Gynecol* 1979:53:25.
9. Srinivasan G, Seeler RA, Tiruvury A, et al: Maternal anticonvulsant therapy and hemorrhagic disease of the newborn. *Obstet Gynecol* 1982;59:250.
10. Little B, Smith OW, Jessiman AG, et al: Hypophysectomy during pregnancy in a patient with cancer of the breast; Case report with hormone studies. *J Clin Endocrinol* 1958;18:425.
11. Rubin R, Brennan RE, Jacobs GB, et al: Cerebral death. *J Med Soc NJ* 1978;75:825.
12. Donaldson JO: *Neurology of Pregnancy*. Philadelphia, The WB Saunders Co. 1978, p 267.
13. Young BK, Katz M, Klein SA: Pregnancy after spinal cord injury: Altered maternal and fetal response to labor. *Obstet Gynecol* 1983; 62:59–63.
14. Aminoff MJ: Neurological disorders and pregnancy. *Am J Obstet Gynecol* 1978;132:325.
15. Comarr AE, Virgil MS: Sexual counseling among male and female patients with spinal cord and/or cauda equina injury. *Am J Phys Med* 1978;57:215.
16. Mandelli M, Morelli, PL, Nordio S, et al: Placental transfer of diazepam and disposition in the newborn. *Clin Pharm Ther* 1975; 17:564.
17. Massey EW, Cefalo RC: Neuropathies of pregnancy. *Obstet Gynecol Surv* 1979;34:89.

CHAPTER 14

UROLOGICAL TRAUMA IN PREGNANCY

HABIB ANWAR
MANUEL FERNANDES
JOSEPH SEEBODE

Urologic trauma is not common in pregnancy. When it does occur, its management can be difficult. Occasionally, the life of the fetus and the pregnant woman are both in danger. The variety of trauma in pregnancy is similar to that in nonpregnant women. Blunt trauma, stab wounds, gunshot wounds, and accidental or intentional acts of violence all could cause urologic trauma.

The symptoms of urologic injury are also similar to those in nonpregnant patients, but often the physical findings are not as obvious. It is important to understand the physiologic and anatomical changes that occur in the genitourinary tract during pregnancy[1] in order to evaluate urological trauma properly.

One of the more common physiologic changes during pregnancy is known as the physiologic hydronephrosis of pregnancy. This occurs most commonly on the right side and almost always begins above the brim of the pelvis. The pathophysiology of this change is not very clear. Hormonal imbalance, compression by the uterus, and diminished ureteral peristalsis have been implicated in this phenomenon. Hypertrophy of the longitudinal sheath muscles especially at the lower end of the ureter (Waldeyer's sheath) or an enlarged uterus per se could be the causative factor for this physiologic change.

The dilation of the left ureter is less common, and this is because the overlying sigmoid protects and cushions the left ureter. Not only is the right ureter dilated more often, but it also shows more deviation. Also, it is important to mention that the right ureter crosses the iliac vessels almost at a right angle, whereas the left ureter descends parallel to them.

In rare cases, an infectious process may be responsible for the hydroureter and hydronephrosis. In the presence of infection, the normal involution process, which is usually 1 month, will be delayed, and occasionally it might take more than eight weeks before the ureters return to their normal size. Renal excretion is prolonged during pregnancy, and this progressively worsens as the pregnancy advances. This fact should be kept in mind when one performs an excretory urogram on a pregnant woman, because 5- or even 10-minute films might not be of diagnostic value. Therefore, it is preferable to obtain one film 20 to 30 minutes after the injection of contrast medium. This also reduces x-ray exposure.

Hypotonicity of the bladder during pregnancy has been documented. Increased vascularity, hypertrophy of the musculature, and edema of the bladder wall have been documented by microscopic studies. The capacity of the bladder progressively increases with advancing pregnancy. Sometimes the bladder can retain twice its normal capacity. Hormonal imbalance is one of the multiple factors responsible for the hypotonicity of the bladder. Mechanical factors such as a retroverted uterus, tumors, cervical fibroids, and uterine prolapse will definitely play a role in overdistention and secondary hypotonicity of the bladder.

Ovarian vein syndrome or pelvic brim syndrome is another entity that is found in pregnant women. Clark in 1964[2] described this syndrome, explaining that the dilation of the right ureter is due to compression by an enlarged crossing ovarian vein. Although this syndrome and its role as an obstructing factor are controversial, several reports indicate its existence and reveal postoperative disappearance of dilation of the ureter after excising the right ovarian vein. Dykhuizen and Roberts[3] explained the pathogenesis of obstruction of the ureter to be secondary to encasement in a common sheath with the right ovarian vein.

RENAL TRAUMA

Microscopic hematuria or gross hematuria will often be detected in patients with moderate to severe renal injuries. The degree of hematuria does not correlate with the extent of the injury. A drip infusion excretory urogram is mandatory for the initial diagnosis of renal injury in order to reveal the site of the trauma and bleeding. It may also point out the presence or absence of the contralateral kidney, something that must always be determined before deciding to save or remove a damaged kidney. The drip infusion pyelography is a preferred method of pyelography which is 70% to 98% accurate when associated with tomography. A normal nephrographic phase will indicate an intact vascular pedicle. On the 30-minute film, the outline of the kidney and ureter will be well visualized. Whenever adequate information is obtained with one film, further exposure of a pregnant woman to x-rays should be avoided. When a major renal injury is suspected, renal angiography should be considered prior to surgical intervention.[4]

In managing a renal injury in the pregnant woman, the general principles for treatment of any multiple trauma patient should be followed. In the pregnant patient who has sustained multiple injuries, including renal trauma, the order of treatment must be dictated by the severity of the injury. Shock due to massive bleeding, associated with rupture of the liver or spleen, would dictate that these injuries be managed first. However, it is possible that severe hemorrhage can also occur with severe kidney lacerations.

Minor renal injury, such as a small laceration with extravasation of urine, is managed conservatively. The patient should be confined to bed with careful observation, and intravenous fluid or increased oral fluid intake is recommended. A dipstick of urine should be done at least twice to evaluate microscopic hematuria. Any sudden bleeding will be detected by checking the hematocrit at least daily.

In pregnant patients with massive renal injury with extensive extravasation, a nephrectomy may be considered if it is known that the contralateral kidney is intact and functioning well. Injury to a solitary kidney should be treated more conservatively, and all possible efforts should be used to preserve that kidney.

Emergency renal exploration is usually accomplished through a midline incision, regardless of the side of the injury, even in the pregnant patient. Other viscera can be examined, and associated injuries can be managed accordingly. Drainage of the renal bed should be maintained by a penrose or sump tube drain for 48 to 72 hours.

If the kidney damage is confined to the upper or lower pole only, a partial nephrectomy is recommended. The renal capsule should be preserved, and the damaged renal parenchyma should be excised. The calices, major arteries, and the veins must be suture ligated. At the end of the procedure, the capsule should be sutured tightly over the excised pole. It is important to avoid nonabsorbable suture materials when operating on the urinary tract. Occasionally, the use of gelfoam or other fibrogenic materials will aid in hemostasis.

SPONTANEOUS INJURIES OF THE GENITOURINARY TRACT

Rare incidences of spontaneous injuries of the kidney, bladder, and retroperitoneal space have been reported. Occasionally there may have been minor trauma. These possibilities, although rare, should be kept in mind when treating a pregnant woman with shock or severe abdominal pain.

Spontaneous bleeding into a retroperitoneal space may occur in hemophiliacs or in patients who are on anticoagulant therapy. Rupture of a renal tumor, ectopic pregnancy, arteriosclerotic aneurysms, and pyelonephritis are all causes of retroperitoneal hemorrhage.

Spontaneous rupture of the kidney in the pregnant woman is an unusual and uncommon complication that may happen in a previously diseased kidney. Rupture may involve the renal parenchyma or the renal pelvis. Predisposing factors for rupture include hydronephrosis, chronic pyelonephritis, tumors or stones in the pelvis, polycystic kidney disease, and tuberculosis. Hydronephrosis has been responsible for the majority of the cases.

Extrusion of the fetus into the bladder from a ruptured uterus is an extremely uncommon disaster that can occur during pregnancy. The lower uterine segment is anatomically very close to the bladder. A laceration into this area could extend easily into the bladder.[5] Previous prolonged labor or pelvic surgery may initiate the formation of scar tissue between the bladder and the lower uterine segment, causing firm adherence of these two organs. This facilitates the extension of a uterine rupture into the bladder.

The signs and symptoms of spontaneous genitourinary injuries may be deceiving. Gross hematuria is not common. Although pain is a persistent finding, shock results only after a massive hemorrhage. An abdominal mass is present if extravasation or bleeding is confined to anatomic barriers. Chronic extravasation from a small rupture may be unrecognized for a considerable length of time. This may be responsible for a perinephric abscess.

When spontaneous injuries are suspected in a pregnant woman, emergency diagnostic and therapeutic steps should be taken as soon as possible. Intravenous urogram, cystogram, computerized tomography scan, ultrasound, and a renal scan may be used to obtain or confirm the diagnosis.

The treatment of a ruptured bladder associated with the pregnant uterus is surgical exploration. Delivery or termination of pregnancy should be performed. The bladder should be repaired in two layers, and a suprapubic catheter should be inserted for better drainage. Rupture of the kidney is managed by a nephrectomy, providing the contralateral kidney is intact and functioning. Treating a rupture of the renal pelvis requires the correction of the obstruction at the ureteropelvic junction and closure of the renal pelvis with 3-0 or 4-0 chromic catgut and adequate drainage.

SPONTANEOUS PERIPELVIC EXTRAVASATION OF URINE

Spontaneous extravasation of urine in the hilus of the kidney has been reported in pregnant women. Usually it happens at term when mechanical obstruction of the ureter at the pelvic brim is at its maximum. The right ureter, as mentioned above, is more often affected in the pelvic brim obstructing mechanism. The clinical picture might be mistaken for pyelonephritis. Limited urography, ultrasound, computerized tomography scanning, and renal scan and urine cultures could be used to rule out other pathology such as infection or obstruction due to a stone. Prompt diagnosis and treatment are mandatory to avoid urinoma, secondary retroperitoneal fibrosis, and perinephric abscess. Spontaneous delivery or caesarean section should be considered as soon as the diagnosis is made.[6]

URETERAL INJURY

Isolated traumatic ureteral injury is rare. Over 95% of all ureteral injuries are caused by a gunshot wound. Although microscopic hematuria is a persistent finding, occasionally a complete avulsion of the ureter will not show any red blood cells in the urine. Infusion intravenous pyelogram and retrograde ureteropyelogram will disclose the extent and the level of injury. Stab wounds of the abdomen rarely damage the ureter. Severe decelerating blunt trauma may avulse the ureter from the renal pelvis. Surgical injuries of the ureter commonly occur during difficult hysterectomy, pelvic, and retroperitoneal surgeries.

At the time of repair of the ureter, it is important to note any effect of a high-velocity missile on the tissue surrounding the injured area. A wide debridement is imperative for the repair of such an injury. End-to-end anastomosis after adequate excision is the treatment of choice for most ureteral injuries. A ureteral stent can be used to ensure the continuity of the ureter. If the ureter is injured in the vicinity of the bladder, a reimplantation with an antirefluxing technique is usually preferred. Repair of a ureteral injury with extensive loss of its lower segment requires a Boari bladder flap with antireflux reimplantation of the ureter into this bladder flap. In this procedure, the ureter is directly reimplanted into the bladder which has been sutured to the psoas muscle. Transureteroureterostomy is another method of ureteral repair. The upper part of the impaired ureter is anastomosed to the contralateral ureter. This procedure should be avoided in patients with a malignancy in the genitourinary tract or a history of stone formation.

PELVIC FRACTURE AND BLADDER RUPTURE

A careful history and physical examination will usually reveal a bladder injury associated with pelvic fracture. The lack of urine after inserting a Foley catheter in a patient with radiologic evidence of pelvic bone fracture will facilitate the diagnosis of bladder injury. A stress cystogram utilizing only two films should be done to document any extravasation. This will also differentiate between extraperitoneal or intraperitoneal rupture.[5] Intraperitoneal rupture will show contrast in between the loops of bowel, the extraperitoneal rupture usually is seen in the form of a teardrop with a wisp of extravasated contrast. Sometimes the fracture of pelvis is associated with urethral injury, and a Foley catheter cannot be passed into the bladder. If so, percutaneous suprapubic cystostomy can be performed for temporary drainage of the bladder. The definitive surgery for the repair of the urethra should be scheduled for a later date when the exploration can be performed. Repair of the bladder and any additional injuries to the intraperitoneal viscera should be undertaken at that time.

PELVIC SURGERY AND IATROGENIC GENITOURINARY TRAUMA

Most major elective surgery should be postponed until the end of pregnancy. If pelvic surgery, caesarean section, or hysterectomy is done on a pregnant woman, the possibilities of genitourinary complications should not be overlooked.

The types of injuries that are encountered during surgery are bladder laceration, ureteral laceration, ureteral ligation, ureterovaginal fistula, urethrovaginal fistula, and vesicovaginal fistula.

Postoperatively, a cystogram and retrograde ureteropyelogram will aid in recognizing the level and extent of injury. At surgery, intravenous administration of indigo carmine will establish the diagnosis.

If a ureteral injury such as complete or partial transection or ligation occurs in the vicinity of the bladder, a ureteroneocystostomy should be performed. Results, using this approach, are superior to any other method. Occasionally, a deligation of the ureter is acceptable, if it is noted during operation and the ureter is not ischemic. If kinks and strictures due to previous surgery have involved the ureters, ureterolysis with or without splinting should be performed. Recognition and repair of a bladder injury is not difficult. Repair usually results in complete recovery. A two-layer closure with absorbable suture is required, and a Foley catheter or suprapubic drainage is used. Ureterovaginal fistulas are managed temporarily by inserting a ureteral stent and covering with antibiotics. About 15% of these will close spontaneously.

With careful and thorough management, a successful outcome can be predicted in most urologic trauma, whether it be in the pregnant or the nonpregnant patient.

REFERENCES

1. Fainstat T: Ureteral dilation in pregnancy. A Review. *Surg Gynecol Obstet* 1963;18:845.
2. Clark JC: The right ovarian vein syndrome, in *Emmett-Wittens Clinical Urography* ed 3. Philadelphia, The WB Saunders Co, 1971, pp 1997–2007.
3. Dykhuizen RF, Roberts JA: The ovarian vein syndrome. *Surg Gynecol Obstet* 1970;130:443–52.
4. Koskela E, Kairalouma MI, Ala-Ketola L et al: Immediate surgical treatment of major renal trauma. *Annals Chir Gynaecol* 1977; 66:144.
5. Montie J: Bladder injuries. *Urol Clin North Am* 1977;4:59.

SUGGESTED READINGS

1. Carlton CE Jr: Injuries of the kidney and ureter, in Harrison, et al (eds): *Campbell's Urology*. Philadelphia, The WB Saunders Co, 1978, pp 881–905.
2. Mattingly RF, Friedrich EG: Difficult hysterectomy. *So Clin Obstet Gynecol* 1972;15:788.
3. McConnell JD, Wilkerson MD, Peters PC: Rupture of the bladder. *The Urol Clin North Am* June 1982;9:2:293.
4. Meares EM Jr: Urologic surgery during pregnancy. *Clin Obstet Gynecol* 1978;21:907.
5. Norman NH, Raghauaiah NV: Spontaneous peripelvic extravasation of urine during pregnancy. *So Med J* 1980;73:809.
6. Read JA, Miller FC, Yeh S, et al: Urinary bladder distention: Effect on labor and uterine activity. *Obstet Gynecol* 1980;56:565.
7. Redman JF: Traumatic renal injury in pregnancy. *J Urol* 1977;118: 845.
8. Rigby MR, MacEwan DW: Urography during pregnancy. *J Can Assoc Radiologist* 1976;27:228.
9. Wesolowski S: Ureteral injuries. *Int Urol Nephrol* 1973;5:39.
10. Aaro LA, Kelalis PP: Spontaneous rupture of the kidney associated with pregnancy. *Am J Obstet Gynecol* 1971;111:270.

CHAPTER 15

BIOMECHANICS OF PREGNANCY

MARLENE J. ADRIAN

One of the major concerns during pregnancy is the adaptability of the person to anatomical and/or physiological changes with respect to pursuing fundamental activities of daily living as well as recreational activities, including sports. This adaptability, or lack thereof, is best understood from the perspective of biomechanics. Biomechanics is that subfield of knowledge which incorporates the study of movement of living bodies, such as the locomotor patterns of walking, jogging, skipping, etc. Biomechanics of pregnancy therefore, may be subdivided into three areas: internal changes, external changes, and functional considerations.

INTERNAL CHANGES

Distinct changes occur throughout the body during pregnancy. Some of these changes are a direct result of changes in the uterus, and others are independent of the uteral changes. Of greatest importance with respect to modifications in motor behavior are the changes in the uterus and the cardiovascular and the musculoskeletal systems.

The uterus is transformed from an approximately 7-cm-long, solid-walled, lightweight tissue to a thin-walled tissue as long as 36 cm and with a 15 to 20 times increase in weight. The entire abdominal wall is stretched, and organs within the cavity are displaced and compressed. In the early weeks of pregnancy these changes are minimal. As the uterus moves from the symphysis pubic level to the umbilical level about five months into the pregnancy and ascends to the subcostal level at nine months the effects of this displacement is noticeable. Concomitant with the displacement is the stress and strain placed upon organs in the abdomen and pelvic cavity. The strains upon organs are a function of the amount of shortening taking place because of compression by the enlarged uterus. The strain upon tissues such as uterus, skin, and muscle is a function of elongations of these tissues. Thus the stresses (force per unit area) are compressive stresses upon organs, including blood vessels, and tensile stresses upon tissues. Primarily the diaphragm, uterus, intestines, stomach, bladder, and inferior vena cava are affected.

Although the diaphragm is elevated approximately 4 cm during late pregnancy the excursion of the diaphragm is not adversely affected during breathing. In 1938, Thomson and Cohen (Buchsbaum) determined that this excursion was increased from 1 to 5 cm.[1] Tidal volume may be increased as much as 40%. The body adapts to the changes caused by pregnancy.

The ureters are displaced laterally and are prone to develop kinks and show marked dilations as early as two or three months into pregnancy. The right ureter is dilated to a greater extent than the left.[2] The bladder is displaced anteriorly and superiorly, partially moving outside the pelvic compartment. During the first two trimesters of pregnancy, the woman may have twice the urine volume as that of a nonpregnant woman. Thus, the pregnant woman may feel bowel discomfort and need to urinate more frequently than the nonpregnant woman.

The abdominal gastrointestinal system is compressed, but only the digestive process in the stomach appears to be affected. The results of a test meal given to women were as follows: At the time that approximately 75% of the test meal had left the stomachs of nonpregnant women, only approximately 56% of the test meal had left the stomachs of pregnant women.[1]

There appear to be no general modifications in the musculoskeletal (including tendon and ligaments) system of pregnant women. The rate of bone tumor and remodeling may, in fact, be enhanced.

Localized changes with respect to the symphysis pubica are pronounced. Ligaments at both the symphysis pubica and sacroiliac joint elongate. As early as the seventh month there is marked widening of the pubis, as much as 0.7 mm.

The distention of the abdominal wall also causes elongations in the muscles of the anterior and lateral walls of the abdomen. The rectus abdominus and internal and external oblique abdominus muscles may be distended to such an extent that they are no longer able to stabilize the lower torso and pelvis. Smooth muscles in the abdomen hypertrophy to protect the intestine from developing kinks.

Increased chest wall elasticity, producing a greater substernal angle and greater anteroposterior diameter, occurs near the end of term. Red blood cell volume, total blood volume, lower viscosity of blood, blood pressure, heart rate, and lower extremity venous pressure all progressively increase during pregnancy. Peripheral resistance to blood flow is generally lowered thus increasing blood flow, whereas compressive stress on the inferior vena cava especially during the supine position may occlude the blood flow in this vessel.[3] The changes in circulatory and respiratory systems may be considered compensatory to supporting physical activity requiring greater energy expenditure than in the nonpregnant state.

EXTERNAL CHANGES

Externally the pregnant woman takes on a different shape. As shown in Figure 15-1, the torso may be increased in diameter to various amounts from the subcostal level to the pelvic brim. In all conditions, the body weight may increase 45 to 225 N (10 to 50 lb.) Since this additional weight is primarily anterior, the force vector representing the line of gravity is directed

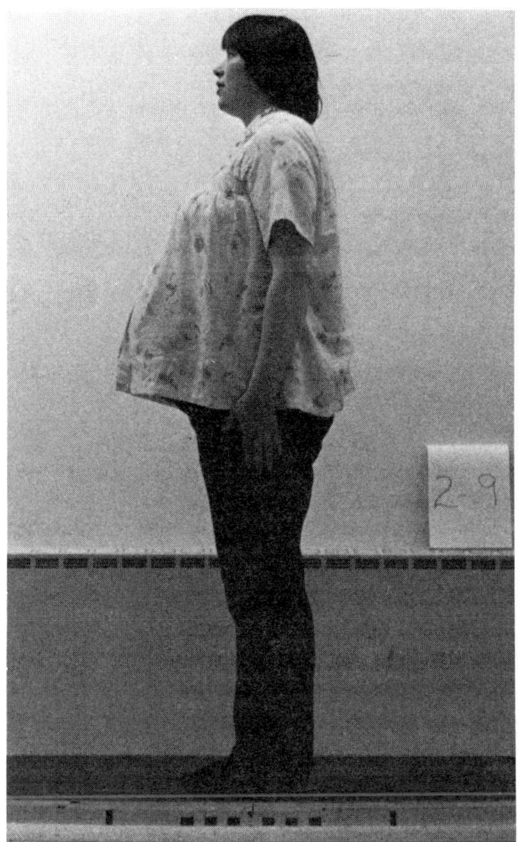

Figure 15-1 Profile of pregnant woman.

downward anterior to the arch of the feet and possibly to the toes of the feet unless compensatory realignment of the body is made. The typical compensation is to lean backward with the upper torso.

During the third trimester, the pregnant woman may be unable to see her feet when standing erect. She may have difficulty in adjusting to the increased weight, tiring more easily and having difficulty in maintaining dynamic balance when walking. If compensatory realignment has been made by leaning backward, she probably will have developed low back pain due to the increased lordotic curvature produced by this balancing technique. Compressive stresses are placed upon the posterior positions of the lumbar vertebrae. The lumbosacral plexus may also be compressed, causing similar low back pain complaints.

The increased weight may also produce pain in the legs and feet during stance and walking. Greater than normal stress may be placed upon the hip, knee, and ankle joints, especially if some malalignment is present.

The position of the center of gravity of the body not only is more anterior, but is higher, and may even be more to the right of the midline of the body than in the nonpregnant condition. This coupled with the additional weight, may produce posture and equilibrium problems. Much like the adolescent experiencing rapid and uneven growth of body parts, the pregnant woman must learn to control and move her new body.

A predisposition to falling is present. Concomitantly, the woman probably becomes more cautious and, with a relatively healthy body, averts falls and broken bones.

FUNCTIONING IN WORK, ACTIVITIES OF DAILY LIVING AND SPORTS

The fitness level and motor activity level of the pregnant woman during her first trimester is a major determinant as the effect of pregnancy upon movement patterns in work, activities of daily living, and sports. If she has been sedentary with a level of fitness barely above the requirements to perform the activity of daily living, the pressures and displacements of the uterus and organs during the first trimester of pregnancy may be disruptive and interfere with normal performance of the activity. The woman with a high level of fitness and motor activity patterns will view these changes as relatively insignificant. Many women will be able to participate in their normal activities of daily living and work, and sport movement patterns without change during their first third of pregnancy. Hormonal changes may adversely influence the movement patterns of pregnant women during these months, but biomechanical considerations usually are not of any significance.[4]

The effect of pregnancy upon movement performance during the second and third trimester is related to weight, position, and activity of the fetus as well as to the fitness and motor activity level of the pregnant woman.

Before the 1960s there was virtually no research concerning the effect of exercise or sports participation upon the pregnant woman or her fetus. Ryan and Allman report that Comenius suggested in the 16th century that pregnant women engage in light exercises to produce lively and vigorous offspring.[5] William and Chir suggest that fitness and physical activity have a beneficial effect on the course of later pregnancy and menopause.[6] Their statement is based upon obstetrical histories of ex-athletes.

Studies by Erdelyi, Zaharieva, and others after 1960 consisted of surveys of athletes in which the data would support the premise that sports participation has no adverse affect upon the pregnant woman or her fetus, and may have none upon the performance as well.[7,9,10]

Newspapers, sports magazines, and books have included articles concerning the many women athletes who have participated in sports competition during pregnancy, even to the last month of pregnancy, without complications.[1,6,7,9-12] For example, June Strove Irwin won a bronze medal in diving while three and one-half months pregnant at the 1952 Olympics. At the Olympic Games in 1956, there were at least 10 pregnant participants including a discus thrower. Some of these women had performed personal bests in National and Olympic competition. One diver won a national championship at six months pregnant. Margaret Court competed in tennis at eight months pregnant and won the Wimbledon after delivery. A woman jockey rode until seven months pregnant. More recently, Robin Beck ran three road races averaging no less than seven minutes per mile while pregnant, the last race was two weeks before delivery.[13] These examples have all been of highly competent athletes in excellent physical status. Testimonials and publicity items are not as readily available for "normal" pregnant women.

Gendel published data on female patients who lacked regular physical activity and lacked strong anterior abdominal musculature.[14] These women complained of lumbar backaches and had chronic fatigue. Prescribed physical activity improved the physical status of all patients by reducing the backache and fatigue.

Certain sports may be contraindicated for pregnant women. Sports in which blows to the abdomen are likely or in which uncontrolled falls will occur should be avoided. Since there is a greater supply of blood in the abdomen in the pregnant state than in the nonpregnant state and the tissues are elongated with tensile stress, the chance of serious hematomia is increased in impact to the abdomen. For example, the sport of foil fencing would place the woman at high risk. In general, the woman is not at high risk in participation in activities of daily living, exercise, or recreational sports. By the latter is meant sports in which the goal is not to win as much as it is to play under control and within submaximal limits. Since the body mass is greater, the energy required for the sports movements will be noticeably greater for a woman during the third trimester than in the first trimester and before pregnancy. Thus the woman will experience fatigue sooner unless she lessens the intensity of participation.

DANGER TO THE FETUS

Danger to the fetus is probably the greatest concern of the woman who is pregnant and is a competitive athlete. The question of how athletic participation and competition should be decreased to assure a healthy birth is an important one. Empirical evidence exists supporting the theory that athletes give birth more quickly, with fewer caesareans, and with fewer abnormalities.[10] Return to athletics also appears to be enhanced during postpregnancy. Woman athletes have set records and performed their best after giving birth. Whether or not these results are a response to several months of forced restricted physical activity, readiness to train more strenuously due to a lesser body weight, or maturity is not known. These improved performances may be considered supporting data for the theory that physically active women, especially athletes, having normal pregnancies experience no deleterious or lasting effects in body function after a first pregnancy. Not enough information concerning multiple pregnancies exists to warrant a similar conclusion.

Caution is given by several doctors, including gynecologists, that strenuous physical activity may be detrimental to the fetus. Two approaches to the determination of the danger level of the activity have been used: 1) demands upon the performer, and 2) hemodynamic changes in mother.

RANKING SYSTEMS

Nicholas has constructed a ranking chart for 61 sports with respect to 21 demands upon the performer. These demands were labeled as performance factors, mental and psychometric factors, and environmental factors and included such items as strength, agility, accuracy, alertness, creativity, and equipment. The higher the score, the less appropriate the sport was considered for the pregnant woman. Ballet, football, and bull fighting were contraindicated, whereas hiking, bridge, and camping were considered to be of little risk. Ranks were based upon subjective ratings of little or no (0), mild (1), moderate (2), and heavy (3) involvement.[12]

A second ranking based upon the motions of walk, run, jump, kick, throw, and stance was also compiled. Again football was highest; likewise, so was basketball. Low rankings were archery, bridge, canoeing, camping, snowmobiling, and deepsea fishing. Motorcycling was assigned a relatively low-risk value as well. Canoeing places a great stress upon the upper body and trunk muscles, including those in the abdomen. Motorcycling and snowmobiling often include collision possibility and "jumps" over uneven terrain. Thus, these ranking systems do not identify all of the risks of all the sports.

A pure biomechanical ranking of sports more clearly might be another means of determining the risk to the fetus and mother. Three factors would need to be identified. 1) High impacts – landings on feet, falls to body parts, collisions with players, equipment. 2) High accelerations – rapid changes in speeds causing movement of the fetus or uterine wall, separation of uteroplacenta junction, or the symphysis pubica. The splits in gymnastics, for example, would be dangerous during the third trimester of pregnancy. 3) High loads – the lifting of heavy weights in which loss of balance could occur, the heavy use of anterior muscles crossing the abdomen resulting in excessive strain.

Although some subjectivity in appraisal of sports is required, more and more biomechanical analyses of actual forces produced during sports are being conducted.[15] In the future, more objective data will be available. At the present time, any one of these three factors (high impacts, high accelerations, high loads) would constitute a danger flag for the sport. The major criterion is whether the body can tolerate the forces produced in the sports situation.

HEMODYNAMIC CHANGES

The second approach is both biomechanically and physiologically based. The hemodynamic changes are in reference to blood flow, volume, and pressure from the uterus to the active muscles during sports participation. It is a well-known fact that blood flow is directed to working muscles during exercise. There have been several studies concerning the physiologic effects of this shift in blood flow upon the fetus. Women have been exercised on a semirecumbent bicycle ergometer according to a graduated program to approximately 80% of maximum.[16] The mean maternal heart rate increased 70 beats per minute,[1] whereas the fetal increase was only 7 beats per minute.[1] No fetal abnormalities in blood pressure or heart rate, such as bradycardia or tachycardia, were noted.

Dressendorfer studied the effects of jogging upon the fetus and pregnant women.[17] The women improved in endurance and maximum oxygen uptake. The fetus showed no abnormalities at exercise rates up to 95% of prepregnancy values. Note that this would represent less than 95% of present value. In both studies, the women were healthy and physically active, though not necessarily athletes.

Uteroplacental insufficiency has been identified by investigators during diagnostic maternal exercise regimens.[18] The women taking part in the test were of a lesser level of fitness than those of the bicycle and jogging studies. Although adverse changes were noted in fetal heart rate in the maternal exercise regimens, some of the investigators here indicated possible previously comprised uteroplacental insufficiencies. The exercise regimen was useful in identifying the existing problem.

The most incriminating data against exercise has been collected using sheep and goats as subjects.[19] Lambs were smaller than normal from four animals exercising for 15 minutes twice daily on a treadmill. The exercise intensity was such that fetal oxygen levels decreased 19% and uterine blood flow decreased 60%. The data of a second study were favorable with respect to treadmill exercises of 30 minutes to 1 hour. These animals were not as forcibly restrained as in the previously mentioned study.[20] Likewise, Clapp indicated that no fetal deterioration occurred in his pregnant sheep until exhaustive exercise.[21]

The conclusion to be drawn from this research on hemodynamic changes in the blood does get shunted away from the uterus during exercise (although one research study in Wisconsin showed no significant changes in sheep exercised to exhaustion).[22] The fetuses of some women will show abnormality in heart rate, and fetuses of well-conditioned athletes will probably show fewer abnormalities of the same percent of maximal exertion.[22]

A last factor, not biomechanics in nature, that needs to be mentioned is the effect of exercise upon the fetal temperature. If blood flow is decreased through the uterus, although exercise causes a rise in rectal temperature the fetus might show an increase in temperature. Not much research has been done to determine exactly what this increase in temperature might be and whether it is detrimental. Speroff recommends not overheating the body during pregnancy and recommends that hot tubs and saunas be avoided in the first trimester. Brief 5-minute exposures to temperatures not exceeding 102°F may be tolerated during the second and third trimesters.

SUMMARY

Empirical evidence and research exist in support of the premise that physical activity and sports generally are beneficial, or at least not deterimental, to the pregnant woman and the fetus. In particular, exercise is beneficial in the adaptation to changes in the position of the center of gravity of the body, increased weight, potential for increased lordosis, and prevention of venous pooling or vena cava occlusion. Stresses and strains upon the abdomen, lumbar spine, and pelvis may produce low back pain and a susceptibility to tissue damage of separation in high-impact, high-acceleration, or high-loading situations. The better the muscular strength of the pregnant woman, the better she will be able to reduce these problems.

The fetus usually is well protected within the abdominal cavity with respect to sports movements. Blood flow and temperature changes, however, may occur under conditions of strenuous exercise which could cause abnormality in the fetus. Therefore, women should exercise and participate in sports to a perceived exertion less than maximum, and possibly less than the perceived comfort zone for them. The avoiding of long periods of overheating and exercise levels of intensity that may cause oxygen shortage to the fetus are rational actions. However, not enough research exists to establish the maximum number of minutes or the numerical level of intensity to guide the pregnant woman. Each woman responds as an individual. What might be safe for one woman may not be safe for another. In general, the more physically fit the woman is at the onset of pregnancy and the maintenance of this level, or the gradual and rational improvement of this level during pregnancy, the better the chances for a healthy child and mother.

REFERENCES

1. Buchbaum HJ: *Trauma in Pregnancy*. Philadelphia, The WB Saunders Co, 1979.
2. Donald I: *Practical Obstetric Problems*. London, Lloyd-Luke Ltd, 1979.
3. Shearman RP: *Human Reproductive Physiology*. Oxford, Blackwell Scientific Publications, 1972.
4. Hale W: Women and sports: Keeping up with female athletes' needs. *Contemporary Obstet Gynecol* 1979;13:85.
5. Ryan AJ, Allman FL: *Sports Medicine*. New York, Academic Press, Inc, 1974.
6. Williams JGP, Chir B: *Medical Aspects of Sport and Physical Fitness*. New York, Pergamon Press, 1965.
7. Erdelyi GJ: Gynecological survey of female athletes. *J Sports Med Phys Fitness* 1962;2:3:174.
8. Zaharieva E: Survey of sportswomen at the Tokyo olympics. *J Sports Med Phys Fitness* 1965;5:215.
9. Zaharieva E: Olympic participation by women. Effects on pregnancy and childbirth. *JAMA* 1972;221:992.
10. Wyrick W: Biophysical perspectives, in Gerber EW, et al (eds): *The American Woman in Sport*. Reading, MA, Addison-Wesley Publishing Co, 1974.
11. Gerber EW, Felshin J, et al: *The American Woman in Sport*. Reading, MA, Addison-Wesley Publishing Co, 1974.
12. Nicholas J: Sports injuries, in Buchsbaum HJ: *Trauma in Pregnancy*. Philadelphia, The WB Saunders Co, 1979.
13. Salmon J: From here to maternity. *Woman's Sports* 1983;44.
14. Gendel ES: Fitness and fatigue in the female. *J Health Phys Ed Rec* 1971;42:53.
15. Cooper J, Adrian M, Glassow R: *Kinesiology*. St. Louis, CV Mosby Co, 1983.

16. Dressendorfer RH, Goodlin RC: Fetal heart rate response to maternal exercise testing. *Physician Sports Med* 1980;8:11:91.
17. Dressendorfer RH: Physical training during pregnancy and lactation. *Physician Sports Med* 1978;6:2:74.
18. Pokorny J, Rous J: The effect of mother's work on fetal heart sounds, in Horsky J, Stembera ZK (eds): *Intrauterine Dangers to the Fetus.* Amsterdam, Excerpta Medica Foundation, 1967, p 354.
19. Pomerance JJ, Gluck L, Lynch VA: Maternal exercise as a screening test for uteroplacental insufficiency. *Obstet Gynecol* 1974;44:383.
20. Hon EH, Wohlgemuth R: The electronic evaluation of fetal heart rate: The effect of maternal exercise. *Am J Obstet Gynecol* 1961; 81:361.
21. Speroff L: Can exercise cause problems in pregnancy and menstruation? *Contemp Obstet Gynecol* 1980;16:57.
22. Stembera ZK, Hodr J: The "exercise test" as early diagnostic aid for fetal distress, in Horsky J, Stembera ZK (eds): *Intrauterine Dangers to the Fetus*. Amsterdam, Excerpta Medica Foundation, 1967, p 349.

INDEX